Healthy Fasting

Margot Hellmiss and Norbert Kriegisch, M.D.

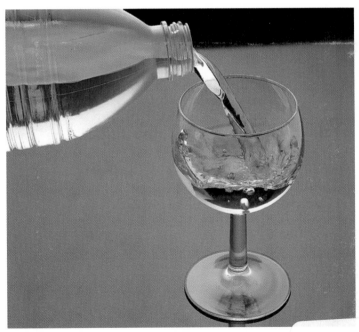

Sterling Publishing Co., Inc.
New York

Library of Congress Cataloging-in-Publication Data

Hellmiss, Margot.
[Schlank und Fit durch gesundes Fasten. English]
Healthy fasting / Margot Hellmiss & Norbert Kriegisch.
p.   cm.
Includes index.
ISBN 0-8069-2027-0
1. Fasting—Health aspects.
I. Kriegisch, Norbert.   II. Title.
RM226.H4413 1999
613.'dc21   99-37579
                        CIP

10 9 8 7 6 5 4 3 2 1

Published by Sterling Publishing
   Company, Inc.
   387 Park Avenue South, New
   York, N.Y. 10016
Originally published in Germany
   under the title *Schlank und Fit
   durch gesundes Fasten* and ©
   1996 by Sudwest Verlag GmbH &
   Co. KG, München
Translation © 1999 by Sterling
   Publishing Company, Inc.
Distributed in Canada by Sterling
   Publishing
   c/o Canadian Manda Group,
   One Atlantic Avenue, Suite 105
   Toronto, Ontario, Canada
   M6K 3E7
Distributed in Great Britain and
   Europe by Cassell PLC
   Wellington House, 125 Strand,
   London WC2R 0BB, England
Distributed in Australia by Capricorn
   Link (Australia) Pty Ltd.
   P.O. Box 6651,
   Baulkham Hills, Business Centre,
   NSW 2153, Australia
*Manufactured in the United States of
America*
All rights reserved

Sterling ISBN 0-8069-2027-0

Contents

A Day of Fasting as Prevention

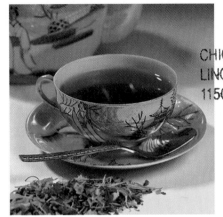

Herbal tea is an important element of most fasts.

The 10-Day Program

The Post-fast Period

Fresh fruit is well suited to the recovery days.

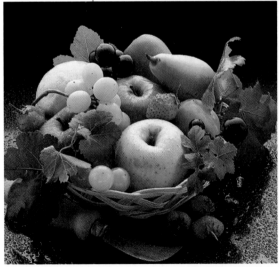

Foreword

A bounty can often become a burden. Fasting can make us aware again of the value of simple things.

We have become accustomed to eating a rich, bountiful diet. Many of us feel that this plenitude enriches our lives. But the danger is that the body and the spirit can slowly grow numb as the desire for more increases. We have become used to finding happiness in abundance, and we are quick to forget that blessings can also be found where there is less. Whoever has fasted knows how exciting the taste of a simple apple can be. The feeling of gratitude for everyday things and the fresh experience that comes after fasting have given many a consumer-weary individual a feeling of happiness that, in spite of our high standard of living, can seem elusive or unfamiliar.

A Few Good Reasons to Fast

There are many reasons that people fast. For instance, some people fast to lose weight or to maintain their ideal weight. But weight loss is only a secondary benefit. What is of primary importance is that fasting purifies the body—it detoxifies, making tissues younger—and "cleans house" not only for the body but also for the spiritual inner life. Our spiritual existence depends more on our eating habits than we think.

Eating a large meal late at night can result in considerable discomfort the next morning. Food is not properly digested during the night. It produces a wide range of fermented toxins in the colon, and these can affect our moods adversely. In such a case, eating earlier and less can be sufficient to put us in a better mood the next day. A fast can do much more—for both the mind and the body.

Different Methods from Which to Choose

In this book, you will find precise instructions, along with tips and advice, for a 10-day fasting program. We also introduce you to programs for only one day, a weekend, and a month. You can choose among different methods, such as juice, tea-juice, milk-bread, whey, and porridge fasts.

Fasting makes us happy, for both body and spirit are cleansed.

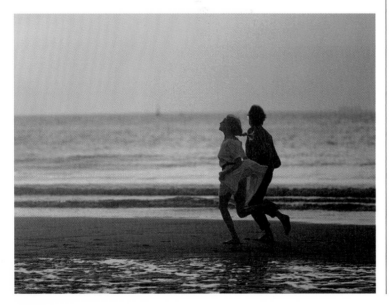

Whether you have just completed a day of fasting or an entire fasting program, you will be amazed by how good you will feel afterward.

What You Should Know about Fasting

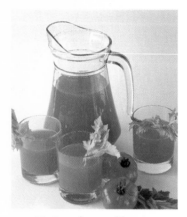

Fruit and vegetable juices are essential elements of many fasts.

Fasting Is Not Starving

Contrary to what some people think, fasting is by no means the equivalent of starving. When people are starving, they want food that they don't have. For most people who are starving, the specter of starvation looms at the end of this involuntary situation.

Fasting, in contrast to starvation, is the voluntary renunciation of nourishment. The time span of fasting can normally be mastered without experiencing a terrible hunger.

Fasting doesn't mean that all consumption is taboo. On the contrary, during a fast, we need to drink a great deal (herbal tea, mineral water, and diluted fruit and vegetable juices), in order to give the body the vitamins and the minerals that it needs and to stimulate the expulsion of toxins by the kidneys. Fasting therefore means drinking.

During a fast, we abstain from consuming true sustenance. But there are even exceptions to this rule. For example, the F. X. Mayr and Schroth methods permit eating bread.

Fasting is a self-evident part of our lives. We eat during the day and fast at night. Our bodies need this natural fast in order to metabolize the day's food.

Fasting and Performance

When fasting, the body acquires the needed energy from reserves. Every healthy person has sufficient reserves to maintain energy even during a relatively long fast. The fat cells are, especially, reservoirs of energy; therefore, the weight loss during a fast shows how much of these reserves were used and turned into energy.

In addition, during a fast, the body has a greater energy capacity, because it doesn't need to spend any energy on digestion. The amount of energy usually required for digestion can be measured by how tired a large meal makes us. It's common knowledge that having a full stomach is not a condition very well suited to studying and no athlete competes after consuming a lavish three-course meal.

The Swedish Fast March

Eleven members of the Swedish Vegetarian Society began their renowned fast march on August 1, 1954. They walked 312 miles (520 kilometers) from Göteborg to Stockholm, arriving on August 10. Often walking through pouring rain, they covered some 30 miles (50 kilometers) a day.

They did without any substantial food and drank only 3 quarts, or liters, of water and some fruit juice each day. Each of the men lost between 17.6 and 22 pounds (8 and 10 kilograms) during this period. But when the walkers arrived in Stockholm, they were in good spirits and still incredibly chipper. All the participants of the fast march were taken to a hospital where they were examined by doctors and given clean bills of health.

It's not necessary to impose extreme limitations on

During a fast, the body transforms energy reserves into power. This process is known as "nourishment from within."

During a fast, it's important to be as active as possible to maintain healthy circulation.

yourself during a fast. Over the course of a fast, people can go about their normal activities (with the exception of heavy labor). Exercise is, in fact, recommended. However, research has shown that people who fast sometimes experience passing concentration lapses or circulation problems. Such apparently harmless conditions can present problems on certain jobs. If you drive a truck or a taxi, for example, you should not fast while working.

Fasting—an Overview

Going over the following points will help you understand what a fast can mean for you.

What You Can Expect during a Fast

▨ Forgoing substantial sustenance
▨ Nourishing yourself from within, from the bodyns own reserves
▨ Drinking a great deal of herbal tea, fruit and vegetable juices, vegetable broth, and water
▨ Forgoing such toxins as alcohol, nicotine, black tea, and coffee
▨ A spiritual high, which comes from a feeling of lightness and can be traced in part to the melting pounds and your pride in your accomplishment
▨ Stimulating evacuation: through the colon (with Epsom salts), through the kidneys (by drinking), through the skin (through movement and sweating), and possibly also through homeopathic remedies
▨ Finding your center through a refined perception of your physical and spiritual surroundings

▧ Physical activity

What You Shouldn't Expect during a Fast

▧ Hunger. Normally slight feelings of hunger cease after the second or third day of a fast. After this point, the body has adjusted to fasting. Hunger should not be confused with the desire to eat.

▧ Bad moods. Most fasting days are, with the exception of the rare crisis day, spent in a somewhat euphoric mood.

▧ A reduced performance. A lower intake of calories will not lessen your performance. On the contrary, fasting enables us to think more clearly and often enhances our performance.

Who Should Fast?

A period of fasting is beneficial for every healthy human being. Fasting is, however, especially recommended for conditions arising from excessive nourishment (which is when more food is eaten than energy is spent). Such conditions include the following:

▧ Joint problems, rheumatic disorders
▧ High cholesterol, liver, or uric acid levels
▧ High blood pressure
▧ Stomach disorders, heartburn
▧ High acidity
▧ Shortness of breath, feeling bloated, being overweight
▧ Bad breath
▧ Problems with hair or nails
▧ Problem skin
▧ Bloated skin, spongy hips, sagging breasts

By means of purging and detoxifying the body, fasting achieves a healing effect. It prevents disease and extends life expectancy.

Such conditions as bloated skin, lethargy, and irritability are often signs of an improper or too rich diet.

■ Digestive disorders
■ Cold sweats
■ Bad moods, irritability, aggressiveness, tendency to complain

Fasts can also benefit people who suffer from the pressures of living in a world dominated by consumerism, as well as people with addictions (with the exception of anorexia, and in the event of a difficult withdrawal), those who tend to be forgetful and unfocused and whose libido is low, those who have lost a sense of the value of life's simpler things, or whoever seeks heightened spiritual and human experiences.

What Fasting Can Accomplish

■ It extends a person's life expectancy.
■ It improves spiritual abilities.
■ It makes the body younger.
■ It heals many disorders.
■ It accelerates the production of new cells.
■ It improves the digestion of nutriments in the body.
■ It stimulates the glands and hormone production.
■ It improves one's performance.
■ It makes tissues younger and skin taut.

■ It purges metabolic waste and toxins.
■ It strengthens the healing powers of the body.
■ It reinvigorates the heart and circulation.
■ It normalizes blood pressure, fat levels, blood sugar, and uric acid.
■ It purifies the body of buildup in the arteries, joints, and tendons, as well as in the liver, the gallbladder, and the colon.
■ It leads to weight loss.
■ It strengthens the body's immune system and natural defenses.

A Short History of Fasting

Fasting as Medical Therapy

Fasting as a method for treating or preventing illness is probably as old as humankind. The Germanic tribes regularly set aside days on which to fast. According to Herodotus, a Greek historian from the fifth century B.C., the ancient Egyptians fasted once a month because they recognized that too much food is damaging.

The famous physicians Hippocrates (460–375 B.C.) and Paracelsus (1493–1541) prescribed fasts for all kinds of ailments. It is also well known that the Spartans kept strict fasting periods, thereby training their bodies to be especially productive.

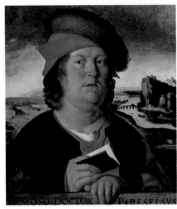

Theophrastus Bombastus von Hohenheim, also known as Paracelsus, a Swiss alchemist and physician

Fluctuations in Fasting Popularity

Up until the end of the eighteenth century, fasting was a popular medical therapy. According to the notes of Alfons Ferrus, who practiced medicine in the eighteenth century, slow and impassive people find fasting easiest whereas those people readily irritated and quick to become angry find fasting more difficult. In around 1840, Osbeck, a Swedish professor, popularized his under-nourishment diet for treating illness. The Swedish government commended him for his efforts.

During the nineteenth century, the age of the Industrial Revolution, technology and science moved

For so-called primitive peoples and in all religions, fasting is a way of maintaining the optimal functioning of both body and mind.

into the foreground and fasting went the way of so many ancient things in the modern world. Doctors forgot about fasting. New, chemically produced medicines and modern machines made it appear old-fashioned.

The Pathfinders of Modern Curative Fasting

Tanner and Edward Hooker Dewey (1840–1904), both American doctors, re-popularized fasting in the United States in the second half of the nineteenth century. They count as among the pathfinders of modern methods of fasting. Dr. Dewey, from Meadville, Pennsylvania, sought out alternative methods of treatment that were focused on the whole human being and not on isolated symptoms. He discovered that through fasting he could achieve the best results for healing various disorders. He especially recommended the morning fast for slightly overweight patients and patients with metabolic problems.

In the German-speaking world, patients have been medically treated through fasts since the beginning of the twentieth century. Dr. F. X. Mayr (1875–1965) and Dr. O. Buchinger (1878–1966) were the first to scientifically study the effects of fasting and worked for its validation among their colleagues.

The Work of Dr. Otto Buchinger

Dr. Otto Buchinger, Sr., is a pioneer in the field of medical fasting. He developed one of the most tried-and-true methods of fasting: the tea-juice fast.

In 1935, Buchinger wrote *Curative Fasting and Its Helpful Methods* (*Heilfasten und seine Hilfsmethoden*), a book in which he established the principles of fasting

The morning fast according to Dr. Dewey: Breakfast consists of a glass of diluted fruit juice along with a cup of coffee or tea. A slightly earlier lunch than usual counts as the first meal of the day.

therapy and made them accessible to his medical colleagues. In addition, he developed guidelines for healthy people who wished to fast at home.

The idea of curing various disorders through the elimination of nutriments came to him after his own experience with a serious illness.

Buchinger's Own Battle with Illness

A case of recurring tonsillitis led to Buchinger's entire body being attacked by the infection, including the colon, the liver, the gallbladder, and the joints. The medical community was unable to help.

Buchinger's condition worsened considerably and finally became life-threatening. Eventually, he could no longer perform his duties as General Physician of the Marines and was discharged as an invalid in 1918 at the age of 40.

Remembering Ancient Remedies

In this difficult time and with his last reserves of energy, Buchinger searched through medical books for a solution. He came upon a report by an American doctor who had treated a similar hopeless case some 40 years before.

The patient was a young girl who was suffering from an infection that had spread to her entire body. Her condition finally improved when the attending physician stopped all food and medicine and administered only water to her. After about a month, this terminally ill patient, for whom all other doctors had given up hope, recovered fully.

Dr. Otto Buchinger became a staunch defender of fasting when he experienced its healing powers firsthand.

Whoever has once experienced the benefits of fasting will fast again and again.

Significant Healing Success

Buchinger immediately underwent a three-month fast treatment under Dr. Gustav Riedlin in Freiburg. After that, his condition improved considerably, and soon he could work again. Following further treatments, he was cured completely.

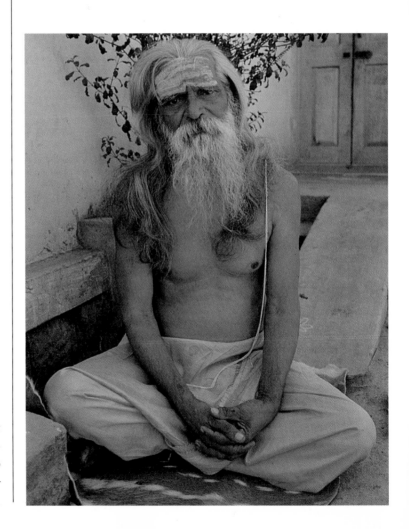

In India even today, there are many people who practice week-long religious fasts. They give up food in order to meditate better and focus more on their faith.

After this experience, he prescribed fasts on an increasing basis for his patients, and in 1920 he opened up his own fasting clinic in Bad Pyrmont in Central Germany.

Religious Fasting

Since ancient times, fasting has been an important dictate in all the major religions. Because fasting requires an act of willpower, it is viewed as a victory of mind over body. Anyone who fasts overcomes physical needs and the desire for worldly pleasures, which is the declared aim of many faiths.

In addition, most religions attribute great significance to the mystical search for inner knowledge. Believers who practice meditation also often fast to purify both body and spirit. This can lead to mental highs and profound spiritual experiences that would otherwise be unattainable.

All major religions see in fasting a path to spiritual experience and inner knowledge.

Fasting Customs in the Islamic World

The Arab prophet and founder of the Islamic faith, Muhammad (570–632), taught: "Prayer brings us halfway to God, fasting takes us to the gateway of heaven." Muslims today still go without food or drink from dawn to dusk during the month of Ramadan in the spring. Smoking is banned as well.

According to the Koran, the holy book of the Muslims, the faithful should make a pilgrimage at least once in their lives to Mecca, the birthplace of Muhammad. The trip is undertaken while fasting. The pilgrims must travel without food for three days

Siddhartha Gautama, the founder of Buddhism, said, "When my flesh disappears, my soul becomes brighter, my spirit more alive in wisdom and truth." In search of spiritual insight, he is said to have nourished himself for six years on grass and seeds.

on their way to the holy site and for seven days on their way back.

Asceticism in Hinduism and Buddhism

In the Vedas, the religious texts of Hinduism, which were written many centuries ago, is the injunction for Indian ascetics to take in their nourishment as if they were consuming medicine. Siddhartha Gautama, the Buddha, or "the awakened one" (560–480 B.C.), following this decree, lived for six years on only grass and seeds.

Fasting in Judaism and Christianity

In the Old and New Testaments of the Bible, fasting often comes up as a means of purification. Moses, the prophet of the Old Testament, fasted for 40 days on Mount Horeb. Jesus also fasted for 40 days in the desert. One of the early founders of the Christian Church, John Chrysostom, wrote: "Fasting is the soul's nourishment, it reins in language and seals one's lips, it tames desire and calms the choleric temperament. It awakens consciousness, renders the body docile, dispels nightly dreams, cures headaches and strengthens the eyes."

Days of fasting were found regularly on the Christian calendar. People fasted before Easter as an act of humility and contrition and in preparation for the coming celebration. Fridays were also days of fasting, on which meat or alcohol, for example, were forbidden (the law of abstinence).

Today, among Catholics, there are just two days of fasting before Easter: Ash Wednesday and Good

Fast—the Word

The word "fast" comes from the Middle High German *vaste,* which means firm, because whoever fasts must hold "firmly" to its rules. The German word *Fastnacht* (Middle High German *vastnaht*) originates from fast. This is the night before the fast that begins on Ash Wednesday.

Friday. On these days, Catholics between the ages of 21 and 60 who are healthy are supposed to fast. They are, however, permitted to eat one main meal and two snacks (without meat) during this time. Protestants, on the other hand, do not set aside specific days for fasting.

Jews still fast traditionally on the holiday of Yom Kippur, also called the Day of Atonement.

Fasting among "Primitive People"

In one of his books, Dr. Ralph Bircher, a physician, reported on the situation faced by the Hunzas, a tribe of some 10,000 people living in a Himalayan valley cut off from the rest of the world.

As with many so-called primitive peoples, the Hunzas had no way of storing food and their agriculture wasn't sufficient to tide them over through an entire year. As a result, they had to fast in early spring until the first barley was ready to be harvested in early summer. Sometimes this fasting period lasted two months. The Hunzas didn't become sick or weak during this period, as might be expected, but continued

Based on his study of the Hunzas, Dr. Bircher was able to show how healthy it is to nourish oneself fully for periods and then to abstain from food.

to work vigorously in the harsh climate. These people normally had no need for doctors—or for police, for that matter, because they coexisted peacefully.

Consequences of "Civilization"

Dr. Bircher also found that nutrition influences social behavior to a considerable degree.

With the encroachment of so-called civilization, the Hunzas lost the need to fast. Now that they could store flour, sugar, and canned goods, there was enough to eat year round. Unexpectedly, the Hunzas began to suffer from a wide range of ailments: cavities, diabetes, obesity, digestive problems, stomach and gallbladder diseases—disorders caused by a poor diet. Struck by the epidemic scale of these ailments, the Hunzas soon began to develop asocial behavior, and outside help was required to maintain order. Suddenly these once healthy and peaceful people needed doctors and police in their isolated valley.

Fasting in the Animal World?

We cannot speak properly of animals fasting, because fasting requires the voluntary decision to abstain from food. Animals do, however, go through periods in which for different reasons they get by without sustenance.

Animals abstain from food instinctively when they are sick. Their bodies need all their energy to fight the disease, and digestion places a high demand for energy on the body.

Many animals have to go without food when its availability is limited, which is mostly the case in the winter. The bear, the hedgehog, and the marmot hibernate during the winter, living from the fat reserves gained over the summer and the fall. When they wake up in the spring, they have lost half of their body weight. Other animals, such as mountain goats, chamois, deer, and wolves, all of which do not hibernate, are also forced to eat less depending on the season.

High Performance Despite a Lack of Nutrition

For deer and chamois, the period of fighting between males for the female occurs during the time of shortage. Although they eat nothing over the entire period, the bucks are still in top shape.

Fish and birds also seem most active when they have the least amount to eat. Salmon do not eat while heading upstream. And some migratory birds can fly for thousands of miles without pecking even the smallest grain.

Animals don't eat when they are sick. This allows the body to focus all its energy on fighting the disease.

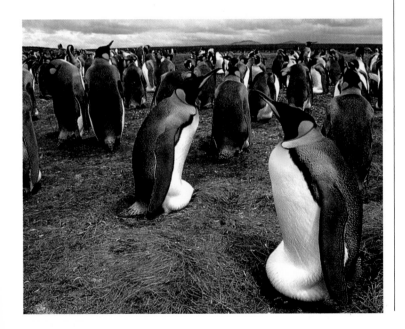

The male emperor penguin doesn't eat for almost nine weeks while incubating its egg, surviving also in spite of the chilling cold of the Antarctic winter. These resourceful birds keep warm by huddling together.

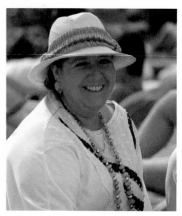

Nutritional slipups in our society often lead to obesity.

**"You turn to medicine and refrain from fasting, as if you could find a better way to heal."
(Ambrosius I, 254 B.C.)**

Medical Aspects of Fasting

Fasting as a Path to a Healthier Way of Life

From a medical perspective, fasting can be seen as a means of eliminating bad eating habits. People who have experienced the effects of fasting on their own body will be more aware of how they nourish themselves in the future. We cannot emphasize this enough. The so-called ailments of leisure, such as obesity, high blood pressure, and hardening of the arteries, which can lead to a heart attack or a stroke, are for the most part the result of a poor diet. Gout, rheumatism, and indigestion, like so many other disorders, are also the consequence of poor eating habits. People who generally eat foods that are too high in fat, sugar, or salt or too rich in protein, or people who just overeat, are the ones at risk here. A fast can bring about a significant change in these people.

Becoming Sensitive to What You Eat

A new attitude is not merely the consequence of the ability to say no that comes with the territory in fasting, but it also results from becoming more sensitive to fatty, sweet, salty, or rich meals. In the days after a fast, that huge serving of pork chops will look less inviting than before—not to mention that they will be quite difficult for the body to digest.

Getting Rid of Bad Habits

The new sensitivity associated with fasting is not just limited to eating. Because the energy from digestion is freed up, we are able to concentrate better on other things. Our awareness of our own body becomes greater, and, at the same time, the spiritual life takes on more significance. During a fast, we become aware of the necessity of staying healthy. A fast can help people to give up a number of undesirable addictions, such as smoking and drinking or even drug abuse. With a fast, all of this disease-inducing behavior is swept away.

Fasting—a Natural Healing Process

Fasting is known as a natural healing process, because it stimulates the body's own capacity to heal. The physician Paracelsus (1493–1541) spoke of activating the "doctor inside," or our own healing nature. This was his motto: *Natura sanat, medicus curat!* ("Nature heals, the doctor helps!").

One of the best examples of the body's ability to heal itself is when we have a feverish cold or flu. Liquids, not food, are the order of the day here. The body, not having to spend energy on digestion, can recover much easier this way.

Fasting rejuvenates the body's natural ability to heal. It is a natural process of healing.

Purging and Detoxification

During a fast, the body purges itself of waste and toxins. Fasting protects us from the effects of both being stored over long periods in the body. We can thus see fasting as a preventive measure performed before the onset of more serious conditions.

The Body "Cleans House"

During a fast, the reserves in the bloodstream, the fatty tissue, and the joints are used for energy. Nothing of value escapes the body.

Before the body attacks its own reserves during a fast, it first uses up the remainder of the nutrients in the blood. During this phase, particles are removed from the bloodstream that would otherwise collect there. The body either uses this material for energy or expels it. The bloodstream is thus the first part of the body to experience relief, as constricted vessels expand. The blood-sugar and fat levels also return to normal. Sometimes, however, it is too late for the hardened blood vessels.

The purging outcome of a fast affects more than the blood—the purifying effects can also be found in the body's fatty tissue, the joints, the lungs, the skin, and, of course, throughout the entire digestive tract. On some fast days, this purification can lead to a slight headache or nausea. The reason for such so-called fast crises has to do with the evacuation of the waste and the toxins. The liver and the kidneys are overwhelmed briefly in their work as the primary detoxifiers. However, this shouldn't be any cause for concern, and you can alleviate the discomfort by

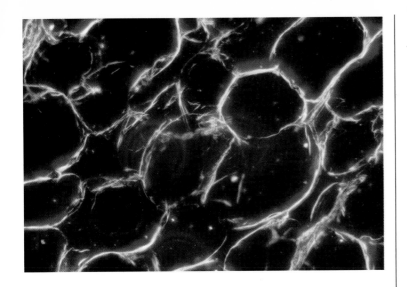

Over the course of a fast, the body falls back on its fat cells for energy. This releases toxins that have built up in these cells.

drinking lots of liquids, which stimulate the toxins' flight from the body.

Digestive Toxins

Digestion produces toxins, such as cresol and fusel alcohol. A healthy person who eats right can expect his or her liver to dispose of these toxins. If, however, the lining of the colon has become irritated through years of bad eating habits, hard spots will form in the lining's folds, poisoning the body at an increasing rate.

This can lead to intestinal autointoxication, whereby the colon poisons itself. The following can be the effects:

■ Headaches
■ Anxiety, irritability, lethargy

Drink, drink, drink—this is the first command of a fast. But even when you are not fasting, you should drink a lot. Your kidneys and entire body will be grateful.

■ Sweating, heart palpitations

■ Pain in the joints

■ Dangerous constriction of the blood vessels

Poisons in the colon can pollute the entire body. This autointoxication (self-pollution) can lead over time to serious illness.

In such cases, fasting can almost perform miracles, especially when accompanied by a colon-cleansing salt (Epsom or Glauber) or an enema. This purifies the colon and spares the rest of the body from constant contamination. Many people who have fasted report that, after several days or even weeks of fasting, unexpected evacuations still occur, proving that the harmful condition has just cleared up.

Avoiding Digestive Residues

During a fast, increasing amounts of toxin are released from the fat cells that are under attack by the body in its search for energy reserves. A large portion of these toxins leaves the body through the colon's mucous membrane. Under normal dietary conditions, they are then discharged with the ballast from the colon. This ballast is lacking during a fast. However, if the waste products remain in the colon, they can pollute the body just like the digestive residues. Therefore, a colon cleansing is highly recommended during a fast in order to stimulate the process of evacuation.

Environmental Toxins

Fasting will also release environmental toxins that have attached themselves to protein in the body's tissues. Toxins, such as DDT, and heavy metals, like mercury, lead, and cadmium, will be discharged by fasting.

In the case of heavy-metal poisoning, the toxins are released from the fat cells. For this reason, any fasting under these conditions should be accompanied by an evacuation therapy (for example, chlorella).

The one thing we know for certain about this process is that it releases undesirable toxins from the fat cells. This includes metabolic waste as well as deposits from the environment. Many of these toxins are consumed in food. The liver makes the toxins as harmless as possible through, for instance, attaching them to amino acids. Fasting is thus a much needed period of rest, allowing the whole body to breathe deeply and recover.

A swollen tongue and the often pungent perspiration during a fast are indicators of the body's increased efforts to detoxify itself.

General Detoxification

During a fast, one's urine contains increased levels of toxins, such as indican and phenol. Pungent sweat and a swollen tongue are also indicators of the widespread detoxification taking place in the body.

The skin around the area of the kidneys and the bladder and also around the colon is one of the most important means of the body's evacuation. The countless sweat glands of the skin expel the poisons, and this can lead to the bathwater or the laundry taking on a brownish tinge.

Tip
While brushing your teeth, be sure to also firmly brush your tongue to remove any film that may have accumulated there during the period of fasting.

Important!

Most of us consume about 15 grams, or 1 tablespoon, of table salt on a daily basis, which is far more than the 3 grams a day that are needed. Ham, canned vegetables, bread, and sausage all usually have high levels of salt. The kidneys cannot process the amount of sodium chloride contained in so much salt, and, as a result, the body can suffer real damage.

The Link between Blood Pressure and Table Salt

People with a propensity toward high blood pressure need to watch their intake of table salt. An excess of salt raises blood pressure and can be one of the causes of a heart attack or a stroke.

The salt discharge is especially high on the first days of a fast. The blood pressure decreases once the salt level in the body has fallen, as long as there is no serious kidney or heart disease or thyroid imbalance.

People who have eaten a diet high in salt often lose up to a couple of pounds (a kilogram) a day during the first days of a fast, because salt causes the body to retain water. After a few days, the weight loss diminishes as the body's salt content drops to a normal level.

Be Careful with Table Salt!

Whether you fast or not, the following applies to you if you have high blood pressure:

■ Use as little table salt as possible!

■ Flavor food with herbs instead of salt.

■ Abstain from salt-laden hams, sausages, and canned vegetables.

■ Eat foods rich in potassium, which is the chemical counterpart to salt. It is found in fresh fruit and vegetables.

Nourishment from Within

Carbohydrate, the Energy Booster

Our most important source of energy is carbohydrates, such as sugar and starch. Semolina, rice, flour, potatoes, and legumes are rich in carbohydrates. We can think of carbohydrates as fuel, because they maintain the body; this is in contrast to protein and fat, from which the body is constructed.

The body transforms most of the carbohydrates directly into energy during digestion. This is called "burning" calories, because oxygen is combined during this process with the carbohydrate molecules. The warmth we feel after eating shows that a type of combustion has actually occurred.

Gaining Energy from the Fat Cells

A portion of the carbohydrates is not burned by the body but stored as reserves. Some 10½ to 14 ounces (300 to 400 grams) are stored in the muscles and the liver. However, these reserves are relatively small and can only sustain a person over a couple of days. An alternate energy source is the body's fat. If we consume more carbohydrate than we need, the body transforms it into fat. It is stored in the fat cells and can be tapped when necessary. There is enough energy stored in the body's fat cells to last a healthy person for weeks without a further intake of carbohydrates.

Carbohydrates are the fuel for the body. In their absence, the body resorts to its reserves, the fat cells.

Why Hunger Fades

This is what takes place during a fast:

■ On the first day, the body still has carbohydrate reserves that it can draw upon for energy.

■ As soon as these reserves have been depleted, the body switches over to a secondary source of energy, the fat cells. This process is known as "nourishing from within."

■ Once the system of internal nourishment has been activated, the early pangs of hunger disappear.

■ Because of this change in the metabolic process, most people find it easier to eat nothing than to eat small amounts. The reintroduction of new carbohydrates disturbs the system of internal nourishment.

■ Each fast makes the change from external to internal systems easier, causing fasting to become less arduous over time.

Hunger pangs are the body's way of signaling its need for its normal ration of carbohydrates. These pains vanish as soon as the body has switched over to its backup system.

The Limits of Self-reliance

In a healthy person, the body's energy reserves can last up to 60 to 80 days. After that, the person can die. However, some exceptions have been reported, such as fasts of 200 days after which no serious damage was found, barring radical losses in weight and energy. A member of the Sikhs fasted 204 days for religious reasons; he subsisted on only water and broth. In January 1995 when he ended his fast, he had lost half his weight—otherwise, he was in good health.

Such exceptions should not, however, be viewed as endorsements for extreme fasting. For medical reasons, extended fasting must be strictly avoided, because it can deplete the body's vital reserves. Moreover, the body needs many years to fully recover from such an assault.

Activity Is Essential

In addition to the fat cells, the protein reserves play a role in the body's search for energy during a fast. A complex series of events in the liver and the kidneys leads to the transformation of protein into carbohydrates that can be used by the body for energy. Alanine, an amino acid, is just one of the chemicals produced in the liver during this process.

Alanine is found in the body's muscles, but only during exercise. Sports, light physical labor, or at least a brisk walk help to maintain energy during a fast.

Outdoor activity in the fresh air can also be good for our moods and can distract us from our hunger. Too little activity during a fast, on the other hand, can lead to poor circulation, which can create further problems.

Protein also supplies energy during a fast. Exercise releases the chemicals necessary for its transformation into carbohydrates.

Losing Weight

How Much Weight Will I Lose?

The longer a fast lasts, the more weight we lose. This is true, at least, for the total days, if not for day-to-day weight loss. As a fast progresses, the weight loss becomes increasingly negligible. The first days are the most significant. Over the days that follow, the daily weight loss is only half to a third of what it was in the beginning. Some days there will even be little or no weight loss.

The exact figures as to how much a person can lose in ounces (grams) per day vary according to the study. We can, however, assume that men will lose about 17½ ounces (500 grams) and women about 14 ounces (400 grams) per day. A daily diet of 200 calories in the form of diluted fruit juice, some honey, and a vegetable broth lowers these figures by some 1¾ ounces (50 grams) a day.

People with less fat are prone to lose less weight than those who are overweight, demonstrating that fasting gets rid of a lot of the body's excess.

Five Percent Reduction

In tapping into its energy reserves, the body begins with the inferior cell material before moving on to the better cells. Fasting is thus a sort of airing out of the body's tissues during which time sick, weak, or surplus cells are purged.

"Seek the angel of fresh air, the angel of water, the angel of sunlight, and the angel of the earth, and invite them to stay with you throughout the fast!" (from the writings of the Essenes, a Jewish community that existed from 150 to 70 B.C.)

Were we to calculate the quantity of inferior cell material in the average body, we would arrive at roughly 5 percent. This translates as follows for a healthy weight-reduction plan:

■ Healthy people of normal weight should fast until they have lost 5 percent of their body weight. For a weight of 154 pounds (70 kilograms), that is 7.7 pounds (3½ kilograms).

■ Overweight people need to choose a percentage depending on their personal needs.

■ However, for both normal and overweight people, the weight loss should never exceed 20 percent of one's body weight.

"Fasting is like being a gifted sculptor who knows how to take areas of fatness and thinness and give them proper form."
(Otto Buchinger, Jr., director of the fasting clinic in Bad Pyrmont)

The Effect on the Acid-Base Level

The Proper pH-Level

■ The pH-level determines whether a solution is, chemically, an acid or alkaline (base).

■ Strong acids, such as hydrochloric acid, can decompose materials, even metals; alkaline, or base, solutions, like soapsuds, can dissolve materials.

The pH-level (p stands for potency, H for hydrogen) tells us about the quantity of electrically charged hydrogen ions in the solution, and thus about its acidic or base quality.

■ Pure spring water is neither acidic nor alkaline and

Important
People whose weight condition requires a loss greater than the recommended 5 percent are advised to seek the medical supervision of a doctor at a fasting clinic. In such cases, a 1,200-calorie diet may be more effective and safer than fasting, because fat returns quickly after fasting when people fall back into old eating patterns.

Did you know that the pH-value of human blood is between 7.38 and 7.44? Blood has slightly alkaline, or base, characteristics.

has a pH-value of 7. Acids have a lower value, bases a higher one.

The pH-level in the human body is determined by:

■ All the body's fluids (blood, lymph, gland secretions, and so forth) that have the same pH-level.

■ The maintenance level of our blood, which lies between 7.38 and 7.44. Below 6.8 and above 7.6 are fatal levels. Such a radical change in the blood's pH-level is almost impossible, because the level is maintained automatically by the body.

Self-regulation of the Body's Acid-Base Levels

The consumption of too many acids from acid-inducing foods, like meat, coffee, alcohol, or sweets, neutralizes the blood's base reserves. The kidneys and the lungs discharge further excess acids to maintain a proper balance.

When these mechanisms no longer suffice, surplus acids are displaced into the body's tissues, creating "acid cells." In the heart, for instance, such a condition can lead to considerable pain and even to a stroke.

The Acid-Regulating Function of the Kidneys and the Lungs

During a fast, the body gets its energy mostly from fat cells (inner nourishment), or more precisely, from the transformation of the acids in fat. As a consequence, the blood and other bodily fluids become more acidic. The number of independent fatty acids in the blood serum climbs, as do other acids that arise during the loss of fat. The kidneys have to deal with these acids, and for that they need 2 to 3 quarts, or liters, of water a day (as much as 5 in the case of very overweight people).

Therefore, people with kidney problems should contact a doctor before fasting. Only the doctor can decide whether or not a fast is in order.

During a fast, there are a number of ways to stimulate the all-important discharge of acids:

■ Fruit and vegetable juices as well as vegetable broth contain valuable nutrients that support the kidneys' discharge of acids.

■ Sweating during exercise or in the sauna helps to regulate the acid base level and generally helps to

There is a sensitive balance between acid and base in the body. The kidneys and the lungs have an important function in maintaining this balance.

detoxify the body during fasting.

■ In addition, physical fitness and breathing exercises are good for the lungs, because they expel carbonic acids to keep the balance. This is also one reason that many people on a fast suddenly feel they can breathe more freely and deeply. This process should be supported.

■ If you wish to use yoga exercises for breathing, it's best to do so with a teacher, because such exercises often affect the body and the mind in a deeper way than we are used to.

The Acids in the Stomach

The stomach hardly has to do any digestive work during a fast. It shrinks and produces fewer salty acids, which are normally required in the decomposition of protein. On the other hand, the stomach is increasingly burdened by acids from the breakdown of fat cells. If you have a very sensitive stomach, you can expect heartburn, burping, or in the worst case a sore stomach.

When the body uses fat for energy, acids are emitted into the body. This is an added burden for the metabolism. Drinking a lot of liquids, sweating, and breathing exercises help the kidneys and the lungs to eliminate these acids.

Warning!

People with a stomach or duodenum ulcer are forbidden to fast. Those who often suffer from stomach pains but want to fast should be examined by a doctor for an ulcer before beginning a fast.

These manifestations are relatively rare for most people who fast and can normally be countered with oatmeal porridge or chamomile tea. When in doubt, a milk-toast diet, such as that of F. X. Mayr, is recommended over a pure juice fast, because the dried bread absorbs the acids in the stomach. Whey and porridge fasts have also proven helpful in such cases.

Fasting and Cancer

According to current scientific knowledge, cancer cannot be cured through fasting. In fact, cancer patients should *not* fast, because it is too demanding.

A recent study by the Institute for Tumor Biology at the University of Vienna does, however, point to the possibility that fasting can hinder the emergence of cancer. This was shown to be the case, at least, in animals. Rats were deprived of food for a period and then treated with chemicals that cause liver cancer. The results of the study showed that the typical growths did not appear or were greatly postponed, and that the risk of liver cancer in these animals was reduced by some 50 percent.

Scientists believe that a fast induces a sort of suicide program in the liver. The cells begin to destroy themselves in the following way: First, the sick cells are destroyed. These are the so-called precancerous cells that produce a tumor. After that, the healthy cells are attacked. Following the three-month fast in

Tip
An overly acidic stomach can be treated with chamomile tea or oatmeal porridge.

Oatmeal porridge
Heat 2 tablespoons oatmeal in ¼ quart, or liter, cold water, and add a pinch of salt. Boil for 2 minutes; add milk.

Tests on animals have shown that fasting can hinder the appearance of cancer.

the study, up to 85 percent of the precancerous cells had died in most of the animals, whereas only 20 percent of the healthy cells had been attacked.

Impeding the Development of Cancer through Fasting

At the Eighth Symposium of the Department of Experimental Cancer Research in Heidelberg, experts indicated that fasting has an effect only when not too many cells are sick—that is, before the appearance of a tumor. Nonetheless, this supports the thesis that fasting is one of the best ways to prevent illness, and even such deadly diseases as cancer.

The opinion also seems to be taking hold within the medical community that too high a calorie intake causes tumors. Fasting, of course, reduces the intake of calories.

Curative Fasting

Fasting not only prevents illness in a holistic way, but it can also lessen or even heal a vast range of diseases and ailments. This is known as curative fasting, in contrast to preventive fasting for healthy people.

Curative fasting is also called "an operation without a knife." It should not be undertaken without medical supervision, and it normally takes place at a fasting clinic.

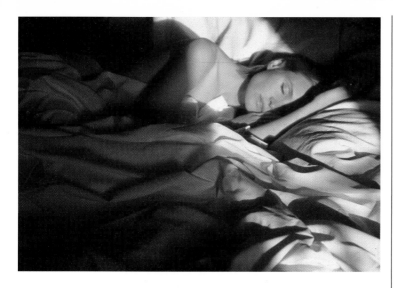

*While we slee[p]...
the body still fun[c]...
"breakfast" is just tha[t]...
breaking of a fast.*

Curative fasting distinguishes itself from fasting for healthy people in two respects:

▪ It lasts at least two to four weeks, entailing a considerably longer period than the maximum of one week of fasting for healthy people. The longer duration is needed to achieve the desired results.

▪ The fasting patient is under a physician's constant supervision and in an emergency can receive the required care.

The overall difference between curative fasting and normal, preventive fasting is, however, minimal. Days of fasting planned by a person at home have a healing effect in cases of digestive problems or high blood-fat levels, for example. Keep in mind that just because a home fast might extend a few days beyond the planned end date, this does not mean that you will require the same treatment as a patient undergoing a curative fast.

Curative and preventive fasting differ in a few respects, but the transition from one form to the other is quite easy.

...we don't eat and ...tions. The word ...—the

Curative fasting takes place under medical supervision and over a period of several weeks.

When Is Curative Fasting Recommended?

Curative fasting, lasting several weeks, is useful in the following cases:

■ Disorders and illnesses throughout the digestive system

■ Colitis and constipation

■ Gas

■ Infections of the stomach and colon linings

■ Some liver conditions, such as a fatty liver or the first signs of liver shrinkage (cirrhosis)

■ Gallbladder infections

■ Cardiovascular disorders

■ Circulation problems, such as arteriosclerosis

■ High blood-fat levels (cholesterol and/or triglyceride)

■ High blood pressure

■ Heart disease linked to closing of the arteries (angina pectoris)

■ Weakness of the heart muscles

■ High risk for heart attack or stroke

■ Infectious skin diseases

■ Eczema, boils, pimples, acne

■ Eye problems, such as running eyes or a sty

■ Illnesses due to allergic reactions

■ Dandruff

■ Rheumatic disorders

■ Bronchial asthma

■ Gout

■ Damaged disks

■ Frequent headaches

■ Depression

Who Shouldn't Fast?

People suffering from the following conditions are not permitted to fast:

■ Consumptive diseases, such as cancer or tuberculosis

■ Thyroid malfunction

■ Psychosis

■ Epilepsy

■ Severe depression

■ Stomach and intestinal ulcers

■ Eating disorders, such as bulimia or anorexia

■ Kidney disease or weakness

Fasting is also banned for people suffering from:

■ Severe undernourishment or starvation

■ Weakness of old age

■ Exhaustion

■ Weak circulation (frequent fainting)

■ Very high blood pressure

■ Feelings of anxiety or of being overwhelmed

In addition, be aware that:

■ Fasting is not advised directly following an operation or a serious illness.

■ Pregnant and nursing women should not fast.

■ Children and teenagers should fast only if they are obese, and the decision should always be their own.

■ Patients under medication need to consult their doctors, because many medications have to be taken on a full stomach.

■ It's a good idea to speak to your doctor first if you are in any way worried about undertaking a fast.

Important
If you take medication regularly, you should consult your physician before beginning a fast.

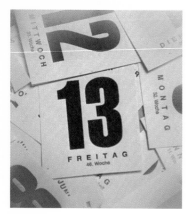

Try setting aside one day a week for fasting, for example, Friday.

Forms of Fasting

How Long Should I Fast?

If you are new to fasting, start with a fast one day a week in which you consume only water, tea, or juice. This stretches the night's normal fasting period over a day. The body will remain switched over on its nocturnal system and continue to draw on its own energy reserves throughout the day.

Fasting One Day a Week

One day of fasting a week does not have the same profound effects of a longer fast. It serves much more as a general means of maintaining good health:

■ Unhealthy conditions, such as high blood-fat content (for example, cholesterol and/or triglyceride), are treated regularly.

■ The heart and other organs, the circulatory system, and the metabolism receive preventive care.

■ High blood pressure is also treated effectively.

■ Weight can be maintained in normal or lost in slightly overweight cases.

Tip
Keep the same day each week for fasting, preferably either Friday or Monday. These days are well suited to fasting, because the meals on the weekend are usually larger than those during the week. On the day of the fast, be sure to drink a lot of liquids and to exercise.

Fasting One Weekend a Month

It's advised for people who work during the week to fast for one weekend a month. The same goes for the weekend fast as for the one-day fast—it's just two days in a row. In this case, too, regularity is more important than frequency.

The weekend is best, because we are normally less busy than during the week and thus better able to concentrate. There is also time for a lot of outdoor activity, relaxing walks, or possibly a light sport such as swimming or bicycling. In addition, we are able to give in to the increased need for sleep.

The 10-Day Program

The 10-day program, which is described in full starting on page 59, starts with a letdown day on which only a light diet is eaten in preparation for the five full days of fasting.

You need at least five days to experience the wonderful effects of fasting. For healthy people, such a period of fasting poses no problem.

In addition, there is a day on which the fast is broken, followed by three recovery days on which the digestive system is reactivated and normal foods are introduced again.

The Long-term Fast

The long-term fast lasts from at least two to four weeks. A fast like this should be taken on only under medical supervision, such as at a fasting clinic, where there is also an atmosphere of camaraderie.

Furthermore, a clinic can offer relaxation and exercise programs, hydrotherapy, massage, and so forth.

Keep a regular day for fasting throughout the year. Or consider fasting every second or third weekend of the month. Consistency is what counts!

When undertaking a long-term fast, it's especially important to break with your daily routine and indulge body, mind, and spirit in a new and pleasing environment.

Different Fasting Methods

Total fasting is often easier than partial fasting, because the body is switched over to the internal energy reserves and doesn't expect external nourishment.

There are different types of fasting, and not every method is right for everyone. For instance, if a particular fast has disagreed with you, you might have chosen the wrong method. Don't be afraid to try a new method the next time. Start with a single day of fasting. Your doctor may be able to advise you regarding which fast to do. You should definitely not switch methods in the middle of a 10-day program. Read about each method here, and let your intuition guide you. You will probably be able to tell right away whether you feel more drawn to milk and toast, to fresh juices, or to a combination tea-juice fast such as Buchinger's.

Full or Partial Programs?

The first four methods introduced here (water, tea, Buchinger's tea-juice, and fresh juice fasts) are regarded as full, or total, fasts, because they completely eliminate caloric intake or reduce it to the minimal form found in juices, broth, and honey.

The other methods (milk-toast, Schroth, and oatmeal fasts) are partial fasts, because the diet is only heavily reduced (bread, whey, oatmeal, or porridge are permitted).

Full Fasts

The Water Fast

■ The water fast is the original form of fasting. It entails drinking 2 to 4 quarts, or liters, of water (without carbonation and sodium-free) a day. In hospitals, this is known as the "zero diet" and is used for weight loss.

Without the supervision of a doctor, this method of fasting should not be carried out longer than a day or two. It is not recommended for a longer period, because the lack of vitamins and minerals can be harmful. At a clinic, the water fast over longer periods is accompanied by supplements, especially vitamin C and vitamins from the B group and the minerals magnesium, potassium, and calcium, which the body needs to stay healthy.

The Tea Fast

■ The tea fast is a natural way of treating a fever. You drink two different herbal teas without sugar or honey three times a day. Mineral water without carbonation should be sufficient to quench your thirst throughout the rest of the day.

As with water fasting, tea fasting entails drinking only calorie-free liquids. You should not do this fast without medical supervision longer than two or three days. People who are elderly or frail are especially advised to take a multivitamin supplement.

Tip
Tea and water fasting are recommended more for individual fast days, because tea and water do not contain any vitamins or minerals.

Important
With both water and tea fasts, an enema or a colon-cleansing glass of Epsom or Glauber salts is highly advised.

The Buchinger Curative Fast (Tea-Juice Fast)

Tip
*The tea-juice fast is especial-
ly well suited to longer
fasting.*

■ The Buchinger curative fast entails consuming 200 to 300 calories in the form of fresh, raw fruit and vegetable juices, vegetable broth, and honey. This method supplies the body with necessary vitamins and minerals. Herbal teas and mineral water can be used to further quench your thirst.

According to Dr. Otto Buchinger, you will be able to achieve a highly effective cleansing and detoxification with this method. And it is better than the classic water fast for treating illness.

This well-proven fast is accompanied by colon cleansings (with Epsom or Glauber salts), physical fitness and relaxation exercises, and hydrotherapy, as well as a step-by-step nutritional recovery program after the treatment.

The Fresh Juice Fast

Tip
*A juice fast is very
appropriate for individual
fast days or for short-term
therapy at home.*

■ The fresh juice fast involves drinking a glass of freshly squeezed fruit or vegetable juice three to five times a day, along with mineral water and herbal tea. Juice fasting supplies the body with many vital materials. The blood takes up these products immediately without overburdening the digestive system.

Potassium, in particular, which appears in high levels in juices, strengthens the evacuation of toxins and acids through the kidneys. The ability of the lungs and the skin to discharge these toxins is also enhanced by juices. In addition, certain herbal teas have special healing powers.

Partial Fasts

The Milk-Bread Fast

The milk-bread fast was developed by F. X. Mayr (1875–1965), an Austrian doctor. On this fast, you are permitted to eat food—bread—with a little milk. The bread should be two to three days old. It is important to chew it thoroughly (approximately 40 times) until it dissolves in your mouth. You can eat until slightly sated. On this fast, you also receive three daily colon cleansings with Epsom salts as well as stomach treatments by a trained Mayr specialist.

The Schroth Fast

Devised by Johann Schroth (1789–1856), a simple farmer and a renowned observer of nature, this fast involves alternating days on which old bread or toast is eaten while drinking a little with days on which a lot is drunk.

■ On Monday, Wednesday, and Friday, the dry days, you are free to eat a lot of bread. In the evening, ⅛ of a quart, or liter, of wine is consumed.

■ Tuesdays and Saturdays are "small drinking days." During the day, you have wine soup, rice, barley, or oatmeal with a lot of bread or toast. In the evening, half a quart, or liter, of wine is consumed.

■ Thursday and Sunday are the "big drinking days." The morning begins with half a quart, or liter, of warm wine or oatmeal soup. Lunch is porridge with plum preserves. Dinner is half a quart, or liter, of wine and bread or toast.

Buchinger's tea-juice fast and Mayr's milk-bread fast are among the most effective fasts you can do.

■ Dry days can involve special or additional food items. Full compresses (Schrottian wraps) are used to stimulate the body's discharge.

The Effect of the Schroth Fast

The Schroth fast lasts at least three weeks and can be undertaken at a clinic.

It has been proven that alternating dry with heavy drinking days has a stronger purifying effect on the body than when, as with other methods, a great deal is drunk consistently. However, what is problematic about this method—and why it's not right for everyone—is that practically wine alone is consumed.

Only people accustomed to drinking in moderation should undertake this method, because those individuals who normally abstain from alcohol can experience negative consequences—as well as become quite drunk.

The Grape (and Other Fruit) Fast

Fasts with grapes and other fruit do not actually count as fasting. They are, however, recommended for a let-down day or weekend in preparation for a fast. Fruit fasts dehydrate the musculature and unburden the circulatory and digestive systems. In addition, fruit contain a lot of vitamins and fiber.

The Whey Fast

The whey fast consists of 1 to 2 quarts, or liters, of dietary whey along with herbal tea and 80 milliliters of fresh herbal juice. Dietary whey from the health food store is quite low in calories but high in vitamins and minerals (especially potassium), valuable proteins, milk sugar, and natural lactic acid.

This fasting method is particularly recommended

for people with sensitive stomachs. It is perfectly suited for individuals with metabolic disorders or colon problems, or those who frequently suffer from constipation and use laxatives. Whey also counteracts a high level of acid in the body, a condition that can arise from eating too much meat.

The Porridge Fast

This is the best method for anyone who suffers from a stomach disorder. It entails eating three portions a day of oatmeal, rice, or linseed porridge. These portions should be swallowed in small amounts. To improve the taste, you can add a little salt, yeast extract, honey, fruit, or vegetable juice. On this fast, you can also drink herbal tea and mineral water.

Whey, or "cheese water," is the watery part of milk that is separated from the curd.

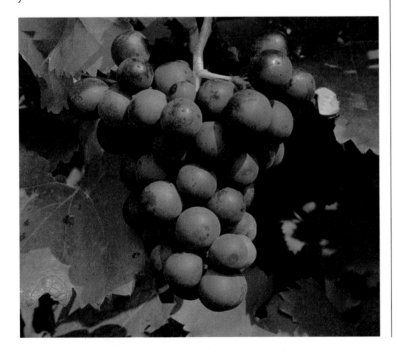

It is especially good for your health in the fall to fast for a day on grapes.

47

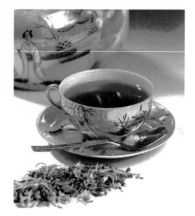

A stylish teacup or an elegant service can make tea fasting fun.

A Day of Fasting as Prevention

Whether you commit to a single day of fasting or to a weekend, the course of the fast remains the same. The day of the fast can even be a workday, although it is better to keep the fasting day free of all obligations.

How the Day Begins

Getting Off to a Good Start

▨ Indulge yourself by turning off the alarm clock the night before and letting yourself sleep until you awaken naturally.

▨ Before leaping out of bed, stay there for a while, stretching. This loosens muscles and joints and heightens your sense of your body.

▨ Follow this stretching with 5 minutes of gymnastics at an open window or, even better, outdoors. Take an "air bath"—undress and spend 15 minutes in a well-ventilated room.

▨ During this time, stimulate your circulation by taking a brush and rubbing it over your body in circular motions always in the direction of the heart until the skin is pink.

▨ Treat your skin to a good body oil afterward. Then climb on the scale and make a note of your weight.

Weigh yourself each morning after going to the toilet; you can be naked, in pajamas, or in a nightshirt—it makes no difference as long as it's consistent.

Bed Exercises

1

Lying on your back, stretch your legs toward the ceiling and peddle for 2 minutes, alternating directions.

2

Extend your legs upward.

3

Then lift and lower the tips of your toes 10 times in a row.

4

Support your rump with your hands, and extend your legs until they are vertical. Count to 20, and then lower them slowly.

■ Now drink a glass of warm water with a teaspoon of colon-cleansing Epsom or Glauber salts. Swallow slowly. Epsom salts (magnesium sulfate) and Glauber salt (sodium sulfate) are natural mineral salts; both dissolve in water and have a gently cleansing effect. They can be found at drugstores.

■ Next, attend to your morning toilet.

■ Remember to finish off a warm bath or shower with a burst of cold water.

Tip
If you don't like the taste of the cleansing salts, an enema, which may be more thorough, can also be used to clean the colon.

The Course of the Day

How to Get Through the Day

■ Drink as much mineral water (sodium-free and not carbonated) as you like during the day, especially if you have additional thirst or feel hungry. You should drink between 2½ to 3 quarts, or liters, a day.

■ Eat each meal at a table that has been set fully, even if the meal is just mineral water, tea, or juice.

Tip
Health food stores and drug-stores sell special fasting teas either loose or in tea bags. These teas contain herbal preparations that facilitate the body's dehydration and removal of acids.

■ If herbal tea is on your fast program, use chamomile, balsamic mint, peppermint, or thyme teas, but don't let them steep more than 2 to 3 minutes. Sugar is not permitted, but honey is okay when specified.

■ Drink the liquid nourishment in small gulps, savoring each mouthful as though you were drinking a fine wine. Try using a spoon. It gives one the feeling of being full quicker.

■ Be sure to get a lot of exercise outdoors. Take a brisk walk, ride your bike, or go for an easy jog for at least half an hour twice during the day. More strenuous sports should not be undertaken during a fast.

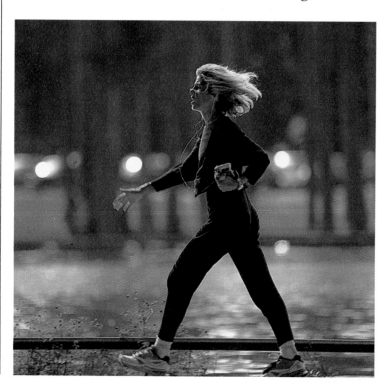

Regular physical activity out of doors, before as well as during a fast, is not only an excellent way of training your body, but it also improves detoxification and the body's process of discharge and prevents circulation problems.

■ Sunbathe, weather allowing.

■ If you are having circulation problems (fainting spells, feelings of weakness, or you easily become tired), drink a cup of black tea with a teaspoonful of honey to stimulate circulation. A glass of buttermilk has the same effect.

■ Allow yourself to rest for an hour or so around noon, and go to bed early (10 P.M. at the latest).

■ Abstain from alcohol and coffee as well as nicotine, if possible. At most, have a cup of black tea in the morning.

■ After fasting, try to eat a lighter, more natural diet.

■ Select your own personal fast day from the following alternatives—the zero-diet, fresh fruit, whey, and juice fasts:

Tip
A footbath under running water stimulates the circulation if it is followed by a final burst of cold water.

The Zero-Diet Fast

■ After waking up, have a glass of mineral water with a teaspoon of Epsom or Glauber salts.

■ For breakfast (and after the morning toilet), have a cup of rosemary tea (which is stimulating) or weak black tea.

■ Over the course of the morning, drink two glasses of mineral water or two cups of herbal tea.

■ Lunch is two glasses of mineral water.

■ Throughout the afternoon, sip a cup of herbal tea (not rosemary tea).

■ In the evening, have two glasses of mineral water.

■ Before going to bed, have a cup of balsamic mint or valerian tea (sleep-inducing).

■ What is permitted on this fast is mineral water (a lot), unsweetened herbal tea, and some black tea.

A side benefit: Even a single day of fasting sharpens our perception of our natural needs.

The Fresh Fruit Fast

Tip
Choose the fruit by the sea-
son: apples, pears, oranges,
plums, or grapes. You can
also combine them. Drink
mineral water immediately
after ending a fruit fast.

■ Upon awakening: A glass of mineral water with a teaspoon of Epsom or Glauber salts

■ Breakfast (after the morning toilet): Fruit, followed by one to two glasses of mineral water

■ During the morning: Fruit, followed by a cup of herbal tea

■ Lunch: Fruit, followed by one to two cups of herbal tea

■ In the afternoon: Fruit and a cup of herbal tea

■ Dinner: Fruit and one to two glasses of mineral water

■ Before bed: A glass of mineral water or a cup of valerian tea without honey

■ What is permitted on this fast is a little more than 2 pounds (1 kilogram) of fruit per day, distributed

Nutritional Value of Various Fruit

Fruit	Calories per 2.2 lbs. (1 Kg)
Apples	500
Bananas	650
Black currants	500
Cherries	520
Grapes	500
Honeydew melon	180
Oranges	390
Peaches	420
Pears	520
Pineapple	300
Plums	590
Strawberries	360
Tangerines	440
Watermelon	110

Apple-Carrot Fast

The following fast has proven to be effective in the event of stomach and colon problems:

1

Eat up to around 3 pounds (1½ kilograms) of apples a day or half that amount mixed with carrots.

2

Eat five portions throughout the day. In the event of diarrhea, finely grate each helping (apples without peels). The high pectin level of the grated apple has a constipating effect. The longer raw fruit and vegetables are left out, the more their value decreases.

3

Drink a few cups of herbal tea with each meal, followed by some mineral water.

over three to five meals, and plenty of mineral water and herbal tea.

The Whey Fast

■ Upon awakening: A glass of mineral water with a teaspoon of Epsom or Glauber salts

■ Breakfast (after the morning toilet): A cup of weak black tea or rosemary tea, sweetened with some honey

■ During the morning: Whey, followed by a glass of fresh fruit juice

■ Lunch: Whey and a cup of green oat tea

■ During the afternoon: Whey and a glass of fresh fruit juice

■ Dinner: Whey and two cups of green oat tea

■ Before bed: A cup of herbal tea (valerian or balsamic mint)

■ What is permitted on this fast is roughly a quart, or liter, of whey (preferably dietary whey from the health food store), which you can divide into several

Tip
Green oat tea can be found at health food stores. It should steep roughly 10 minutes before being filtered.

Tip
The whey must always be kept refrigerated. Drink it in small amounts or, better yet, with a spoon.

servings, along with plenty of sodium-free and non-carbonated mineral water, teas, and some fruit juice.

The Juice Fast

■ Equivalency: 3½ oz. (100 g) of juice is a tenth of a quart, or liter.

■ Upon awakening: A glass of mineral water with a teaspoon of Epsom or Glauber salts, 3½ oz. (100 g) vegetable juice mixed with 1¾ oz. (50 g) herb juice (or 5¼ oz. [150 g] vegetable juice)

■ Breakfast (after the morning toilet): About 2 oz. (60 g) fruit juice

■ During the morning: About 2 oz. (60 g) fruit juice

■ Lunch: 3½ oz. (100 g) vegetable juice mixed with 1¾ oz. (50 g) herb juice (or 5¼ oz. [150 g] vegetable juice)

■ During the afternoon: About 2 oz. (60 g) fruit juice

■ During the evening (no later than 7 P.M.): 3½ (100 g) vegetable juice and about 2 oz. (60 g) fruit juice (do not mix)

■ Before bed: 1¾ oz. (50 g) herbal tea (sleep-inducing tea) and a glass of mineral water

■ What is permitted on this fast is about half a quart, or liter, of fruit, vegetable, and herb juices over three to five servings, some herbal tea, and plenty of mineral water (at least 2 quarts, or liters).

Observe the following guidelines when fasting with juice:

■ The juices must be organic (without preservatives) and unsweetened. It is best to buy them from a health food store.

■ All juices should be mixed 1:1 with mineral water.

Tip
Should you have a sensitive stomach, oatmeal, rice, or linseed porridge can help you digest the juices better.

Tip
If you make your own juices, be sure to use fresh fruit and vegetables each day, otherwise valuable nutrients will be lost.

Fruit Juices and Their Healing Powers

Fruits and Berries	Effect	Vitamins	Minerals
Apples	Relieve diarrhea, acid B6, C, carotene*,	pantothenic acid** Potassium,	phosphorus
Bilberries (whortle-berries)	Prevent diarrhea	C, carotene	Potassium, calcium
Blackberries	Prevent diarrhea, eliminate phlegm	C, carotene	Potassium, calcium
Black currants	Dehydrate, lower blood pressure, boost energy	C, carotene	Potassium, calcium, magnesium
Blueberries	Strengthen immune system, lower fever	C	Potassium, calcium, magnesium, iron
Cherries	Strengthen blood	B6, C, carotene, pan-tothenic acid	Potassium, calcium
Elderberries	Strengthen immune system	C	Potassium, phosphorus
Grapes	Purify, strengthen, and produce blood, dehydrate	A, C	Potassium, sodium
Oranges	Strengthen immune and nervous systems when energy and vit-amin C levels are low	A, B6, C, pantothenic acid	Potassium, calcium
Peaches	Improve skin, detoxify	B6, C, carotene, pan-tothenic acid	Potassium
Pears	Dehydrate, lower blood pressure	A, C	Potassium
Pineapple	Good for skin and eyes	A, C	Potassium
Plums	Stimulate a lazy colon	B1	Potassium
Strawberries	Clean blood, dehy-drate, strengthen nerves	C, carotene	Potassium, calcium

*Carotene forms the rudiments of vitamin A (provitamin A) and is transformed in the body. **Pantothenic acid is water-soluble and one of the B-group vitamins.

The healing powers of fruit and vegetable juices complement the metabolic process optimally during a fast.

Vegetable Juices

Vegetable/Herb	Effect
Artichoke	Stimulates gall flow and detoxifies liver, lowers level of fat in blood
Birch	Dehydrates, diuretic
Carrot	Healing, fights infection, improves skin (e.g., acne) and eyes
Celery	Detoxifies, purges
Dandelion	Dehydrates, detoxifies
Garlic	Prevents the constriction of arteries, lowers blood pressure, fights germs
Hawthorne	Strengthens heart, improves circulation
Horseradish	Diuretic, disinfectant
Juniper	Stimulates joint metabolism (in cases of rheumatism and arthritis)
Onion	Lowers blood pressure
Parsley	Dehydrates, diuretic
Potato	Counters too much acidity in stomach
Radish (black winter radish)	Prevents infection, loosens phlegm, cough suppressant
Sauerkraut	Stimulates digestion
Stinging nettle	Detoxifies, purges
Tomato	Normalizes the digestive system
Watercress	Detoxifies, purges

■ Drink any homemade juices directly after making them. Don't store them, because they lose their nutritional value even after standing out for only 10 minutes.

■ It's up to you which juice you want to use. You can also mix various juices, but don't combine fruit and vegetable juices.

The Porridge Fast

■ Upon awakening: A glass of mineral water with a spoonful of Epsom or Glauber salts

■ Breakfast (after the morning toilet): Porridge and one to two cups of herbal tea

■ During the morning: About 2 oz. (60 g) fruit juice

■ Lunch: Porridge, followed by two glasses of mineral water

■ During the afternoon: Two glasses of mineral water

■ Dinner: Porridge, followed by one to two glasses of mineral water

■ Before bed: A cup of (sleep-inducing) tea

■ What is permitted on this fast is three servings of porridge (oatmeal, linseed, rice, or wheat; see below), seasoned to taste, about 2 oz. (60 g) fruit juice, herbal tea, and plenty of sodium-free, noncarbonated mineral water.

Tip
Porridge fasts are especially well suited to people with stomach disorders. However, if you suffer from a stomach or intestinal ulcer, you should not undertake a fast.

Recipes for Porridge (One Serving)

The four recipes that follow can be used for a porridge fast. Depending on your preference, you can stick with the same type or alternate among recipes.

If you suffer from stomachaches while fasting, a small mouthful of porridge often helps. Prepare a small amount in advance, put it in a thermos to keep it warm, and place it beside your bed so that you can have a soothing drink at night, too, should the need arise.

Oatmeal Porridge

Ingredients: Half a quart, or liter, of water and 3 tablespoons of oatmeal

Instructions: Place the water and the oatmeal in a pot on the stove, and bring to boil. Boil for 5 minutes, and then strain. Season the oatmeal as you like with a pinch of salt, yeast extract, some honey, or fruit or vegetable juice. Eat with a spoon, or drink in very small mouthfuls.

Linseed Porridge

Ingredients: Half a quart, or liter, of water and 2 to 3 tablespoons of finely grated or crushed linseeds

Instructions: Place the linseeds and water in a pot, and boil for 5 minutes. Strain to remove the seeds, and eat with a spoon or drink small amounts. Season the linseed porridge the same way as the oatmeal porridge.

Rice Porridge

Ingredients: Half a quart, or liter, of water and 3 teaspoons of rice

Instructions: Place the rice in water, and bring to a boil. Simmer for 20 minutes on a low flame. Then remove from stove and strain. Season as above and eat in small amounts.

Wheat Porridge

Ingredients: Half a quart, or liter, of water and 3 tablespoons of roughly ground wheat grain

Instructions: Mix the wheat with cold water, and bring to boil. Let cook for 2 minutes, while stirring. Afterward, strain. Season as above, and eat in small amounts.

The 10-Day Program

Introduction

Once you have made the decision to fast, you have already taken the most significant step. Completing a 10-day program is, in comparison, relatively easy. Look forward to the fast as a personal endeavor that ultimately will affect your health, your well-being, and your spiritual life.

Think about how easy fasting can be. The dreaded pangs of hunger will be overcome quickly. It will be a little more difficult to accustom yourself to not chewing during a meal. But undoubtedly, after the fast, you will enjoy a simple meal twice as much as before. Make it clear to yourself exactly what your goals are—this will make it easier to turn the idea of fasting into a reality.

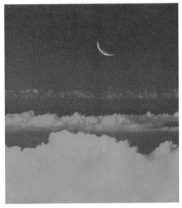

The days before the new moon are the best on which to undertake a fast.

Why Do I Want to Fast?

Mark those boxes that apply to you:

- ■ To take care of my health in general ❏
- ■ To enhance my well-being ❏
- ■ To achieve inner balance ❏
- ■ To keep my weight stable ❏
- ■ To lose weight ❏
- ■ To cure a minor health problem ❏
- ■ To break with bad eating habits ❏
- ■ For religious or spiritual reasons ❏

There are many reasons for fasting. Think about what your own reasons are. This will help to motivate you and see you through to the conclusion.

Important
Don't force yourself to fast.
You have to want to do it.
This is the only way that you
will be able to reach your
goals. By the same token,
don't try to force others to
fast. It's better to lead by
example.

Who Can Undertake This Fast?

Basically, all healthy people can handle the 10-day fast on their own. If you have any doubts about your health, first go to your physician for a checkup.

You should take on the 10-day fast under medical supervision if you:
■ don't feel healthy,
■ are already undergoing medical treatment,
■ are chronically ill, or
■ are on regular medication.

The Right Time

The most favorable time to fast, according to the lunar calendar, is during the days preceding the new moon. The new moon is the best time to end a fast and to make a fresh start.

Many people like to fast in the spring, in order to lose the weight that they have gained during the winter. They want to get back in shape before they get into their bikinis and bathing suits. In addition, a fast during the spring helps the body adjust to the warmer weather, because this switch involves an entire series of metabolic changes.

■ Most people find it more pleasant to fast during a warmer season, as fasting can sometimes bring on chills. Warm weather is also conducive to eating light meals and lots of liquids.

■ According to Dr.Otto Buchinger, people who have a close relationship to nature fast best during the spring, when the opening of buds awakens in them the need to purify and renew both body and spirit.

■ For realistic people—who stand, so to speak, with both feet planted firmly on the earth—the summer is the best time to fast.

■ In the fall, artistically inclined people tend to fast well.

■ The winter, according to Buchinger, is the best time for overweight people to fast, because they have enough nutritional reserves in their bodies to keep from freezing over the cold months.

Fasting and Your Everyday Routine

You can, of course, undertake a fast while working. Some people prefer this, because work provides a distraction from thinking about food and hunger. However, you should be aware that a lack of concentration and irritability can sometimes result. In addition, there will be the culinary temptations of the workplace: the birthday cake, coffee, or lunchtime with colleagues.

■ People whose work involves strenuous physical labor, high levels of concentration, or the use of heavy machinery, and who are directly responsible for the safety of others, such a surgeons, pilots, crane operators, roofers, and bus drivers, should not fast while working.

Set Aside Some Free Time!

If you want to achieve the best results for the body and the mind, it's really to your advantage to sacrifice a few vacation days. As you continue to eat less, your mind will become more clear, and freed from the distracting obligations of your job you will be better able to slow down and focus on your inner self.

Warning
Even healthy people should not fast (total fast) longer than six or, at the most, seven days without medical supervision.

Fasting while continuing to work is usually not a problem, but the experience will be that much more meaningful and intense if you fast during the peace and quiet of a vacation.

How Often Can This Fast Be Done?

It is recommended that the 10-day program be carried out once a year. However, many people prefer to do it twice a year or even more frequently.

With or Without One's Partner?

Fasting is easier if you are not alone. If you can't convince anyone to fast with you, consider looking for fasting courses offered by community colleges, parks, and churches.

Basically, it makes sense to fast with your spouse or partner or with a friend or colleague. The crucial first days of the fast will be that much easier the more support you have. Go out together, or meet in the evenings at the gym.

Community colleges, municipal parks, and churches offer fasting courses. At these nightly meetings, theoretical and practical guidance is provided and personal experiences (as well as problems) are discussed.

In any event, you should inform your family. Let your family know that you might be different from usual. If you normally cook at home, try to make other arrangements. However, after one or two days of fasting, you will find it easier to resist the temptations in the kitchen.

■ In general, it's probably best not to inform anyone in your life who for some reason opposes fasting. Constantly being told that you are ruining your health, look starved, and should eat is an unwanted hindrance to a successful fast.

Grocery List for the Full Fasting Days

The grocery list for the letdown day in preparation for the fast (page 66) should be planned by you, according to the fast you have chosen.

You probably already have these items at home: lemon, honey, black tea, vitamins, wheat germ, table salt, potatoes, and season-ings (bay leaf, juniper, and peppercorns).

You should also have Glauber or Epsom salts, sauerkraut juice, herbal teas (a variety), plenty of mineral water, veg-etables for the fasting soup (celery, parsley, fennel, carrots, and leek), and fresh parsley, as well as fruit, veg-etable, and herbal juices.

Tip
Plan your fast around birth-days, fa ily gatherings, and so forth, leaving at least a week between the end of the fast and the event.

Preparation

You need to do the following before beginning the actual fast:

■ Notify your family.

■ Cancel all other plans and invitations for the week.

■ Find a room or a comfortable spot in which you can retreat, possibly at night as well.

■ Buy the items on the grocery list.

■ Indulge yourself with a bouquet of flowers.

■ Firmly tell yourself that you will complete the fast.

■ Set aside a notebook to be used as a fast diary.

A fast needs to be pre-pared for properly. Not only do you need to plan what to buy, but you also should think about when and how the fast is to be carried out. It's also helpful to think of positive activities to fill the time during the fast as well as to anticipate any problems that might arise.

The Fast Diary

The fast diary is used during a fast to give concrete expression to fleeting thoughts and emotions. Writing will help to give you a sense of clarity.

By keeping a diary, you will gain knowledge apart from that concerning your relationship to food and to your body. Through the process of writing things down, you will discover fears, desires, your position within your family, your relationship to your spouse or partner, and so forth. Let yourself be surprised by what comes up.

The following can be recorded in the fast diary:

■ Your reasons for fasting, your fears and doubts, hopes and desires

■ The daily meal plan with drinks

■ The course of each day, including events, personal impressions, experiences, feelings, and dreams

■ Your weight each day

■ How you are coming to terms with fasting: what you like, what irks you

■ Any problems you may be experiencing

Tip
Use the fast diary to formulate your reasons for, and goal in, undertaking the fast. The more conscious you are of the reasons for your decision, the better you will be able to stick to the fast.

What You Can Expect

■ Eating and drinking by family members
■ Advice from someone who wishes to divert you (perhaps subconsciously) from your goal
■ Possible passing moments of slow circulation

■ Periods of lessened powers of concentration and ability to react (drive carefully!)
■ Sensitivity to loud noises and conflict
■ Slight chill (dress warmly!)
■ Possible heavy sweating

Things to Keep in Mind during a Fast

Positive Thinking

Don't let yourself become preoccupied during a fast with your tax return, relationship troubles, your child's failing grades, illnesses, or other problems. All this distracts from the fast and can be better dealt with afterward when it will appear in a new light.

Drugs

Abstain from alcohol and, if possible, also from nicotine during the fast. Alcohol places a strain on the liver, which has enough to deal with discharging proteins. Caffeine also shouldn't be consumed because of its strong influence on the heartbeat.

Medication

Fasting does not go with medication. People who take pills regularly should fast only under a doctor's supervision.

Secret Snacks

People who eat the wrong foods or too much food during a fast may damage their health, and, of course, they ruin the fast.

Liquid Meals

These are meals consisting of only something to drink. They are, nonetheless, meals. Give yourself time to have these meals as you would a normal meal. Drink small amounts, or use a spoon. Drink more than your thirst demands in between meals.

"Fasting is the strongest appeal to the human being's natural powers of healing and self-rejuvenation, on both a spiritual and corporeal level."
(Dr. Heinz Fahrner, a physician specializing in natural healing and fasting)

The Structure of the Fast

The 10-day program consists of a letdown day in preparation for the fast, five days of fasting, a day for breaking the fast, and three recovery days. This program is based primarily on the proven methods of Dr. Otto Buchinger. Variations are, however, possible.

The Letdown Day

A successful fast should include a letdown day prior to the fast, the fast days, a day for breaking the fast, and recovery days. This structure has proven to be highly effective.

The letdown day is a day for changing gears. Not only do you change what you eat on this day by eating as little as possible, but you make a change, too, in your state of mind. Free yourself, if possible, of all your obligations. Allow yourself to be you. You'll find out that this isn't as simple as it seems. You might actually need a few days for this adjustment, so don't hesitate to begin.

Do what you enjoy, get some exercise, sleep, or meditate. Listen to your body's needs. You might have trouble at first receiving its signals. Read a good book, perhaps one about the positive effects of fasting. Find motivation. Familiarize yourself with the rules of fasting.

Guidelines for eating on the letdown day:

■ Eat simply and lightly. Fruit, raw vegetables, rice, and potatoes (see the meal plans, starting on page 68) should be at the top of the list. Add to these quark (similar to cottage cheese), yogurt, and multigrain bread.

■ Avoid meat, so that the residue of animal protein doesn't remain fermenting in the body.

■ Have a tablespoon of crushed linseeds mixed in a bowl of low-fat yogurt or a glass of buttermilk three times a day. Linseed binds itself to toxins in the colon and acts as a ballast as the body discharges these products.

■ Drink a lot (2½ to 3 quarts, or liters, a day) of noncarbonated mineral water and herbal tea without sugar.

Other points to follow on the letdown day:

■ Eat only when you are truly hungry, not just because it's mealtime.

■ Set the table completely, and eat in peace.

■ Eat slowly and chew thoroughly, laying down your utensils after every bite.

■ Eat only until the first feelings of satiation, and leave the rest on your plate.

■ Drink no more than a cup of black tea or coffee in the morning.

The letdown day should attune your body to the coming days of fasting; it also prepares the colon and the other detoxifying organs.

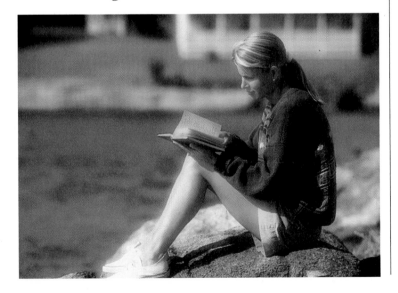

Try something besides television. Listen to music, or read a good book.

For the letdown day preceding the fast, there are five different plans to choose from: fruit, the fresh food diet, rice, potatoes, or the mixed-meal plan.

Tip
Eat a banana in the evening on the fruit day in order to bind the acids.

■ Don't eat between meals, or eat only fruit or raw foods.

■ Go walking for at least half an hour, or find another way to be active outside (tennis, Ping-Pong, jogging).

■ Put yourself mentally in the mood for the coming fast days.

Choose from the following suggested meal plans:

The Fruit Day

■ Morning/noon/evening: Eat 2 to 3 pounds of fruit during the day over the course of three meals.

■ Eat what you like: oranges, apples, pears, figs, bananas, plums, berries, and so forth.

■ Drink mineral water only after some time has passed following the fruit meal.

The Fresh Food Diet

■ Morning: Fruit, fruit salad, or Bircher muesli (see the recipe on the opposite page)

■ Noon/evening: Fresh lettuce salad, with carrot shavings and raw sauerkraut, mixed with oil, lemon, herbs, and spices

The Rice Day

■ Morning: 1¾ oz. (50 g) rice, fermented in milk, without salt or sugar, with cinnamon if you like and diced apple or applesauce without sugar

■ Noon: 1¾ oz. (50 g) rice, fermented in water,

without salt, mixed with crushed tomatoes or carrots and spiced with herbs, and, if you like, oatmeal
■ Evening: 1¾ oz. (50 g) rice, fermented in water, without salt, possibly with cinnamon and diced apple or applesauce without sugar

The Potato Day

In the event of acidic tissue—for example, gout and increased levels of uric acid:
■ Morning: Two to three whole potatoes, freshly cooked on the stove and peeled, spiced with fresh herbs (parsley, dill, cut leek) and some herbal salt substitute
■ Noon: Whole potatoes with herbs (as above), along with oatmeal and steamed vegetables
■ Evening: As in the morning

The Mixed-Meal Plan

■ Morning: Bircher muesli (a Swiss breakfast cereal, see the recipe below)
■ Noon: Fresh fruit and vegetables, cooked potatoes with herbal quark
■ Evening: Fruit or fruit salad with crushed linseed, low-fat yogurt, a piece of toast

Recipe for the Original Bircher Muesli

Ingredients: 2 to 3 tablespoons oats, a container of low-fat yogurt (or a cup of milk), a small apple, 1 teaspoon chopped nuts, 1 teaspoon honey or moist raisins, and 1 teaspoon fresh lemon juice

Tip
For the Bircher muesli, the original muesli by Dr. Bircher, you can choose whatever nuts and types of fruit you like and the oats can be replaced with any whole-grain cereal.

Tip
Plan a treat for yourself for when the fast is over: taking a weekend vacation, going shopping for something new to wear, buying a book that you have always wanted to read.

Instructions: Wash the apple, and grate it with the peel. Mix the yogurt (or milk), the oats, the grated apple, and the chopped nuts in a bowl. Top off with honey or raisins and the fresh lemon juice.

The General Course of the Letdown Day

■ Morning: Weigh yourself right after getting out of bed (with an empty bladder), and write down your weight in the fast diary.

■ Midmorning: Do 30 minutes of brisk walking or light jogging.

■ Noon: Rest 1½ to 2 hours; if you don't want to or can't sleep, try to relax by reading.

■ Afternoon: Do 30 minutes of exercise—for example, brisk walking, light jogging, swimming, or Ping-Pong.

■ Evening: Take a relaxing bath, and read a book about fasting.

The Full Fasting Days

The First Day of Fasting—Letting Go

Tip
If you find that you are experiencing especially sharp hunger pangs, taking the Glauber or Epsom salts solution (salt to water ratio is 1:1) again or having an enema can help.

The first day of fasting starts off with a thorough colon cleansing. The ingestion of Glauber or Epsom salts helps to empty the colon. As a result, the body switches over internally from taking in nutrients to discharging waste and toxins. After the colon cleansing, early feelings of hunger will dissipate. This is the body's signal that the switch has been made.

If you get hungry on the first or second day of the fast, drink some water or a few mouthfuls of buttermilk. Or find a distraction—for example, call a friend, read a book, or take a walk. Keep in mind that your body has what it needs. Open yourself up to the new experience of fasting. You will soon notice everything is basically the way it was before—the only difference is that you are not eating.

The Glauber Salt Method

■ Glauber salt is named after the alchemist Johann Rudolf Glauber (1604–1670), who discovered its effects. It can be found at drugstores.

■ People of average weight should place about 2 tablespoons in half a quart, or liter, of lukewarm water.

■ Those people with constipation or indigestion should use a little more of the Glauber salt.

■ A squirt of lemon improves the taste.

■ Drink the mixture slowly and in small mouthfuls after waking up.

■ Drink some unsweetened peppermint tea or fruit juice to counter the bitter taste.

■ Throughout the morning, you will experience a number of watery bowel movements, so stay near a toilet.

■ Rest afterward with a hot water bottle on your feet.

■ To further stimulate the evacuation of the colon, try drinking a glass of sauerkraut juice, whey, or buttermilk on an empty stomach.

Important
If you are especially sensitive in the stomach or colon areas, you should abstain from taking Glauber salt and have an enema instead.

Tip
Drinking some sauerkraut juice on an empty stomach is another alternative.

The Second Day of Fasting—Eliminating Extra Weight

True hunger is quite rare on the second day of fasting. But what can be difficult is abstaining from food when the fruit bowl or the delicious-looking meal on

Tip
Enemas can also be per-formed at other times, such as during a fast crisis or when hunger gnaws at you.

Colon-Cleansing Plan

Fasting Day	Measure (in the Morning)	Alternative
Day 1	About 2 table-spoons Glauber or Epsom salts	Enema, 1/8 quart (liter) sauerkraut juice, whey, or buttermilk
Day 2	None	None
Day 3	Enema	1/8 quart (liter) sauerkraut juice, whey, or buttermilk or 1 teaspoon Glauber or Epsom salts
Day 4	None	None
Day 5	Enema	Same as for the third day

Tip
Women who normally take a birth-control pill in the morning should wait until three hours after taking the Glauber salt solution. Otherwise, its effectiveness cannot be guaranteed.

the cookbook cover catch our eyes. It isn't hunger that we feel as much as the desire to consume some-thing. This is an important distinction and one that it helps to recognize. However, once we have accepted stopping eating, other consumer-oriented wishes sometimes also disappear. For instance, if your closet is already overflowing, instead of wanting to buy more clothes you might wish to donate a lot of your clothing to charities and make a big break with every-thing. This kind of thinking is not uncommon.

■ People used to drinking black tea or coffee will be more easily tired. Either give in to this urge to sleep or go outdoors and do some exercise to refresh yourself. Coffee really isn't that important! People who are cold should dress warmly.

■ During the first two to three days of fasting, the weight loss is greatest, because the letdown day and the Glauber salt cure dehydrate the body. Losing weight should not, however, be the main reason for fasting. This is more of a side benefit. Detoxifying the body and purging it of waste are much more important, because they eliminate a source of potential illness.

The Third Day of Fasting—Getting Over the Hump

On the third day, like the fifth, the morning begins with a colon-cleansing enema. This removes toxic waste products from the digestive tract, which is important because a bowel movement seldom occurs during a fast. Without such measures, the waste products from the body's tissues that have not metabolized can end up back where they started. Headaches, aching muscles, anxiety, and irritability are signs that such a reverse pollution is taking place.

■ People who don't want to perform an enema should drink ⅛ quart, or liter, of whey, sauerkraut juice, or buttermilk to stimulate the bowels.

■ If that doesn't work, they should try the Epsom or Glauber salts solution, drinking slowly and in small mouthfuls. The other methods (enema, sauerkraut juice, whey, buttermilk) are all preferable to the Epsom and Glauber salts, though, because the salts disturb the normal functioning of the colon. They should thus be used sparingly.

■ This is the day on which you will be able to breeze

A squirt of lemon makes the Glauber salt solution taste better and easier to swallow.

Tip
If you are feeling a little down, don't just lie there in bed. Activity fortifies. Also, try drinking a cup of tea with a teaspoon of honey.

past the grocery store without a problem. You can also probably cook for your family or go with someone to the pizzeria. It feels great to be able to look at everything without needing to have it.

However, on the third day, some people begin to exhibit slight crisis symptoms:

■ Disturbances in vision are the result of less internal pressure on the eyeball. This is nothing serious and will go away.

■ In the event of fainting spells, dashing cold water on the face or the legs or eating half a teaspoon of honey can help.

■ You may feel weak in the legs, and noises can be especially irksome.

Although the first days of the fast can sometimes be critical days, true emergencies arise only after longer periods (two or more weeks). Nonetheless, symptoms of ailments that healed long ago have been known to recur during these days. The body is only now finally overcoming the residue of these ailments. Feelings of depression are also possible and are best countered with activity. A brisk walk outdoors can dispel most morose moods.

The Fourth Day of Fasting—Gains from Abstinence

Tip
It is best to fast until the coating on the tongue disappears. This normally occurs on the fifth day.

By the fourth day, you start to experience nature in a new way. You look at things more closely, your sense of smell is more acute, and you generally feel more alive. You can look at yourself from a distance now, from the outside. You experience yourself with all your strengths and weaknesses. Although you accept yourself the way you are, you may decide to change a

How to Perform an Enema

What You Will Need
■ An irrigator with a water bag, a hose, and an intestinal tube from a drugstore or a medical supply store
■ Lubricant, such as Vaseline
■ Water at body temperature

How It Is Done
■ Fill the water bag with a quart, or liter, of water at body temperature.
■ Hang up the enema bag on the doorknob or a towel rack.
■ Rub the lubricant on the intestinal tube and on the anus.

■ Kneel on one knee, and press down as if having a bowel movement.
■ Insert the intestinal tube carefully into the anus.
■ Now kneel on both knees on the floor, supporting yourself on both elbows.
■ Let the water slowly run from the enema bag.
■ Try to hold in the water for a while.
■ After a few minutes (2 to 5), you will feel the need to evacuate the bowels.
■ Rest for about 20 minutes afterward, with a hot water bottle across your belly to help you relax.

Tip
The devices necessary for an enema can be found at a drugstore.

few things. This is not a contradiction anymore.
■ Your face has changed: It has collected, become more narrow. It even looks older than normal (this will change). Your eyes are larger and have a new brilliance.
■ The coating of your tongue has turned a grayish white.

Tip
The water used in an enema can contain various additional ingredients. For example, for heavy-metal poisoning, use 2 tablespoons of chlorella powder to 1 quart, or liter, of water.

The Fifth Day of Fasting—Renewed Energy and Vitality

Today is the last day of the full fast. You start this day again with an enema. Now you may feel like fasting for another couple of days. You can do this if you want to. The others can go to the farmers' market in the afternoon to shop for breaking the fast and the recovery days. You will see that walking through the market will be easy, and that you will look forward to biting into that apple tomorrow.

The Meal Plan for All Five Days

■ Mornings: Two cups of herbal tea (rosemary, balsamic mint, peppermint, chamomile, or ginseng) with 1 teaspoon honey, or weak black tea with lemon
■ Throughout the morning: Sodium-free, noncarbonated mineral water (at least two glasses)
■ Noon: Half a quart, or liter, of vegetable broth (fasting soup, see page 79) or ⅛ quart, or liter, fresh vegetable juice with the same amount of mineral water (hot or cold)
■ During the afternoon: Two cups of herbal tea with lemon and/or ½ to 1 teaspoon honey

The kidneys need to be thoroughly cleansed during a fast, in order for them to properly discharge the toxins from the body.

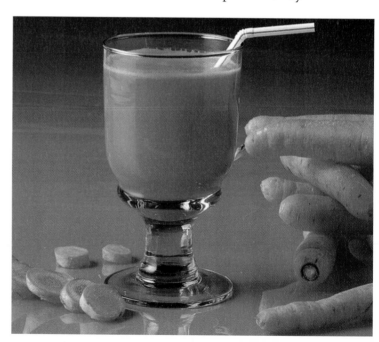

Carrot juice (fresh is best) contains an especially large amount of beta-carotene, the so-called provitamin A, and plenty of vitamin K as well.

Warning!

1	**2**
Instead of this particular meal plan, based on Buchinger, you can plan the five days of the full fast from among the following: ■ Whey fast ■ Pure juice fast ■ Porridge fast The daily meal plans can be found in the chapter "A Day of Fasting as Prevention," starting on page 48.	All the other points of the 10-day program should be applicable regardless of what alternative meal plans you follow. **3** Use the Glauber or Epsom salts and the enemas as described here as well.

▧ Evenings: ⅛ quart, or liter, fruit or vegetable juice, mixed with ⅛ quart, or liter, mineral water (hot or cold), or vegetable broth

Drinks

The liquid meals (following Buchinger) consist of 1 quart, or liter, of fluid. In addition, you should drink mineral water until you reach the recommended daily amount of 2½ to 3 quarts, or liters. During a fast, you need to drink more than your thirst dictates.
▧ The fruit and vegetable juices should always be mixed with water 1:1. You can make them yourself (in a juicer) or have them prepared at the health food store. Freshly made juice should be used immediately, otherwise it loses its nutritional value. If you prefer, you can warm up the juice (don't boil).
▧ People who tend to have trouble with their stomachs should add a teaspoon of linseeds to the glass of juice.
▧ The porridge fast is well suited to individuals

Tip
To avoid having to get up a lot during the night to go to the bathroom, drink most of your daily requirements of liquid before 4 P.M.

Soothing tea for the stomach: Mix chamomile, peppermint, and balsamic mint teas in equal amounts. Sprinkle 1 tablespoon per cup in boiling water, let stand 10 minutes, and strain. Then slowly drink in small mouthfuls.

Herbal Teas and Their Effects

Tea	Effect
Green oat	Reduces uric acid (gout)
Rosemary	General stimulant
Balsamic mint, valerian, orange blossom	Soothing, sleep inducing
Horsetail	Diuretic
Birch leaves, dandelion	Detoxifies
Fennel, caraway	Fights flatulence
Wormwood, gentian root	Stimulates circulatory and digestive systems
Thyme	Relieves cramps
Ribwort	Loosens phlegm
Chamomile, peppermint, balsamic mint	Soothing for the stomach and colon
Elder	Sweat-inducing
Lime flower	Strengthens the immune system
Oak bark	Strengthens the colon, prevents infection
Mallow	Loosens phlegm, prevents infection
Ginseng	Strengthens the immune system, creates balance
Rose hip	Strengthens the immune system
Fennel	Loosens phlegm, fights flatulence
Blueberry, blackberry	Prevents infection

who have sensitive stomachs but want to fast nonetheless. Instructions and recipes for the porridge fast can be found on page 57.

■ In general, your urine should be light (it is darker in the morning, meaning more concentrated, because we usually don't drink during the night). If it is fairly dark, this is an indication that the body's fluids are low and you need to drink more liquids.

Recipe for the Fasting Soup

Vegetable Broth (for Four Portions)

Ingredients: 3½ oz. (100 g) celery bulb, parsley stem, and fennel bulb, 1¾ oz. (50 g) potatoes, 1 oz. (30 g) leek, a small carrot, other vegetables of your choice such as fennel or tomato, a pinch of salt, yeast seasoning, two bay leaves, four juniper berries, and four peppercorns, a quart (liter) water, and freshly chopped parsley

Preparation: Cut the vegetables into small pieces, and add to the cold water. Add seasoning, and bring to a boil. Simmer for 20 to 30 minutes. Strain. Add a little salt and ½ teaspoon yeast seasoning. Top off with parsley.

Suggestions for Things to Do on the Five Full Fasting Days

■ Mornings: Weigh yourself, take an enema on the third and fifth days, do gymnastics or jog, take an air bath, do a dry-brush message, take a hot-and-cold shower.

■ Throughout the morning: Go for a walk, participate in light sports, hike, sunbathe (don't forget the suntan lotion!).

■ Noon: Rest for 1½ to 2 hours in bed (a damp compress helps the liver to do its work), getting up slowly afterward to avoid overwhelming the circulation.

■ During the afternoon: Go for a walk, participate in light sports, hike, ride your bike.

■ Evenings: Read something that is edifying or entertaining, sit quietly in candlelight, meet with others who are fasting to share experiences.

A warm compress on the liver soothes the internal organs, stimulating circulation and thereby intensifying the liver's job of detoxification. You will find instructions for making a liver compress on the next page.

How to Make a Liver Compress

1

You need a flat hot water bottle, hot water, and two towels.

2

The simplest liver compress is the hot water bottle across the liver covered by your blankets.

3

The most effective compress can be accom— plished by placing a moist, warm towel between the hot water bottle and your skin. Place a dry towel on top, and cover yourself well.

4

This stimulates the circulation (40 percent more than normal) and helps the liver to do its work of detoxifying the body.

What Can Occur during the Fast

A Diminished Need for Sleep

Tip

If you are not able to sleep, refrain from taking sleeping pills or other medication. A good way to deal with insomnia is to wash yourself with cold water and climb back into bed without drying yourself off.

It's possible that you will feel more awake than usual at night and have trouble sleeping. Recall the Bible verse "As you fast, so will you awake. Don't complain, use the time."

Instead of turning pointlessly in bed, spend the time meaningfully by reading a book, writing in your fast diary, enjoying quiet music, thinking, practicing yoga, or doing some kind of visualization exercise.

■ Get accustomed to making going to bed a ritual, even when you aren't fasting, a ritual in which the body prepares to glide into the realm of dreams.

These pointers may also be helpful:

■ Don't stay up too late watching television.

■ Go for a short walk in the evening.

■ Air out the bedroom well. The window should also be open at night.

■ Take a brief shower with cold water, or give yourself a cold footbath.

■ Don't cover yourself too warmly.

■ Try not to worry about major problems before going to bed.

■ Think about something that makes you feel good, be positive, and look forward to sleeping.

Tip
Don't go swimming in an unheated outdoor pool during a fast.

Chills

You may get chills frequently during a fast, because the body's ability to keep warm decreases as it looks for energy reserves. The inner heating system has been switched over for a time to an energy-saving system. An old book of fasting tells of the "frigidity of the faster."

■ Put on warm clothes, wrap yourself in a warm blanket in the evening, and lay a hot water bottle across your stomach or feet. These help.

Tip
Give yourself a temperature-raising footbath, and massage the soles of your feet afterward with a lymph lotion.

Bad Breath

Bad breath during fasting is the result of the body discharging toxins. Brush your teeth several times a day, floss, and use mouthwash sparingly. Sucking on a slice of lemon or drinking a mouthful of freshly squeezed lemon juice helps too. Or suck on a piece of sugar-free peppermint candy.

Tip
To eliminate bad breath and improve the taste in your mouth, chew on fresh herbs, such as lemon balm, parsley, thyme, or dill.

Circulation Problems

Circulation problems during a fast are usually caused by having less blood sugar and lower blood pressure. A spoonful of turnip juice, dissolved in hot water, can counter problems with circulation. A cup of weak black tea (not later than 2 P.M., because it interferes with sleeping) with a spoonful of honey, a glass of milk with honey, or a glass of buttermilk can also help.

Warning!
Do not engage in demanding sports during a fast unless you are accustomed to them. Lengthy activities, such as hiking, walking, swimming, and bicycling, are best. Short activities, like sprints or climbing stairs, should be avoided.

Activity and Exercise

Being active is an essential element of fasting. Swimming, dancing, skiing, and hiking help to pump oxygen through the blood, and this stimulates the metabolism, leads to a thorough cleansing of the blood and the tissue, and accelerates the loss of fat.

You will soon discover that physical activity won't tire you but rather will keep you wide awake. As a side benefit, it also helps in the venting of aggressions that sometimes rise to the surface during a fast.

What's more, exercise curbs hunger. Participating in light sports, digging in the garden, or even vigorously cleaning house can make those hunger pangs disappear.

Walking and Hiking

Walking and hiking are ideal forms of exercise, even for people who are not athletic. They utilize the most muscles in the body. You will breathe deeper and strengthen your heart, and even the smallest vessels, the capillaries, will be flushed with blood. In addition, being out of doors in nature stimulates and raises the spirit.

Walking in the Dew

■ Walk through the wet grass barefoot in the morning.
■ Roll your feet in the grass, feeling the moisture and the earth under them.
■ Walk for a while on your toes, then on your heels.
■ Afterward, slip into wool socks with your feet still wet. They will soon be warm.

Outdoor exercise improves the circulation and increases the discharge of toxins through the skin.

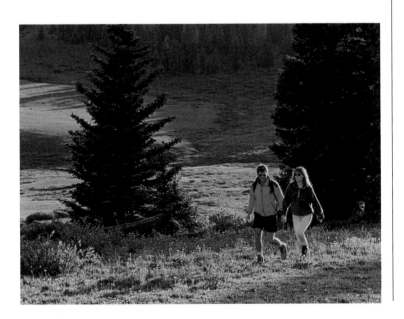

An easy hike in the woods is good for our health and a special pleasure well suited to a fast. It is especially enjoyable in large groups.

Breathing Exercises

Breath is life. Many people, unfortunately, breathe incorrectly or develop anxieties or blocks that impair their breathing, leading to harmful consequences for their health. Through specific breathing exercises, it is possible to reverse these conditions and return to an inner state of balance.

A fast is a good time to get rid of harmful breathing habits with the aid of certain exercises.

Observe the Way You Breathe

■ Sit with your legs crossed or on a chair; your shoulders should be relaxed.
■ Close your eyes.
■ Breathe regularly and evenly, and follow your breath through your body.
■ Feel yourself breathing, but try not to influence it.
■ Feel your chest and abdomen move in and out.

Yoga Breathing Exercise (Pranayama)

■ Sit with your legs crossed or on a chair, keeping your shoulders relaxed and your back straight.
■ With the thumb of your right hand, hold your right nostril closed, and breathe in with the left.
■ Don't try to control your breathing; let yourself breathe naturally.
■ Then, with your middle and ring fingers, hold the left nostril closed, and slowly exhale through the right nostril. You will notice that it takes at least

Tip
It's best to do the exercises outdoors or at an open window.

Tip
The breathing exercises described here can also be done at work. If you do them regularly, you will find that their relaxing effect can be long-lasting.

twice as long to exhale naturally as it does to inhale.

■ Before inhaling, enjoy for a moment the feeling of having let go that comes from exhaling.

■ Breathe like this for as long as it feels comfortable, but don't do it more than three times a day or for more than 5 minutes.

■ You can also do this exercise to relax during a couple of spare minutes at work.

Waiting to Inhale

■ Lie down on your back. Exhale for as long as possible. Count silently in your mind, and each time will be a little longer. Inhaling will be automatic—you won't need to do a thing.

■ Then exhale again for as long as you can, and so forth.

Body and Skin Care

About a third of the body's toxins and waste products are discharged through the skin over the course of a fast. The skin sweats more than usual during a fast, and the result is unpleasant body odor. Proper skin and body care is therefore a necessity when fasting.

Bathe and shower daily, but never in water warmer than 100.4 degrees Fahrenheit (38 degrees Celsius). Because the skin is drier than usual, use a moisturizing cream. Avoid heavily scented or perfumed lotions to spare your heightened sense of smell. Natural, organic products are best.

Toxins are also discharged through the skin. A massage with a dry brush facilitates this process.

The Dry Brush Massage—How It Is Done

What You Need

You need a loofah glove (loofah is a hard, natural sponge) or a natural hair brush.

What You Do

Brush in circular motions and always in the direction of the heart.

Start with the right leg (first the sole of the foot), and then proceed to the left leg, the right arm, the left arm, the back, the belly, the chest (avoid the nipples), and the neck.

The Dry Brush Massage

A dry brush massage can do wonders for your physical well-being, because it:

■ removes dead skin and blemishes,

■ stimulates the glandular, circulatory, and nervous systems,

■ opens pores so that the skin breathes better and can discharge the body's toxins,

■ strengthens circulation and the autonomic nervous system,

■ refreshes you and makes you look younger,

■ strengthens muscles, and,

■ when done with a hot-and-cold shower, strengthens the immune system.

Regularly clean your massage brush with water and hang it out to dry.

Warning!
Don't do the dry brush massage if you have varicose veins or hardened capillaries.

Hot-and-Cold Shower

After giving yourself a dry brush massage, it is recommended to spray down your legs with cold water (for no longer than a minute) or to take a hot-and-cold shower.

■ Shower for 2 to 3 minutes under warm water until the body is well heated.

■ Then shower for 10 to 20 seconds under cold water or water as cold as you can stand.

■ Repeat three times, and finish with a good blast of cold water.

■ Dry off afterward with a coarse hand towel, and massage your skin with lotion (almond, avocado, or orange).

The dry brush massage and the hot-and-cold shower are recommended right after waking up in the morning and before going to bed at night.

A hot-and-cold shower stimulates all the body's systems, especially the glands, improves circulation, and enlivens the skin.

The Day after the Fast and the Recovery Days

Just as important as the fast is breaking the fast and the time for recovery. The body switches back during this time from internal to external nourishment. This process

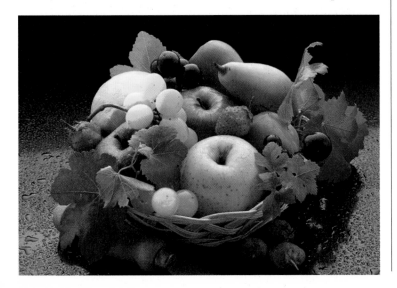

After the strict days of fasting, the fast is finally broken and the recovery days follow. Your first bite into a piece of fresh fruit will be an exquisite joy!

takes longer than the change from eating to fasting. Otto Buchinger, Jr., thus recommends that "the reintroduction of healthy nutrition should take place lovingly and in an intelligent, deliberate, and moderate fashion."

Over the four days following the fast, you will return incrementally to a normal diet, gradually re-activating the colon.

The First Apple

The first real sustenance you will have upon breaking the fast, aside from figs or prunes, is an apple. A simple apple will probably have never tasted better. It contains valuable minerals, and its pectin content stimulates the colon. When you eat this first apple in the morning, include the peel and the seeds.

Rules for the Recovery Days

During the recovery days, it is okay to eat less than prescribed, but not more!

Stop eating as soon as the slightest feeling of being sated sets in.

Alcohol, nicotine, coffee, and sweets are still taboo.

Eat every bite slowly, and chew thoroughly.

Continue to drink mineral water and unsweetened herbal tea.

Stimulating Colon Activity

Eat a teaspoon of finely crushed linseeds with each meal. Mix the seeds with 3 tablespoons of curdled milk and 1 teaspoon of sandwort juice (sweetened with honey).

Linseed contains important fiber that ensures that

"Every fool can fast, but only the wise man knows how to break a fast." (G. B. Shaw, writer, 1856–1950) the digestive system will quickly resume working. In addition, it supplies the body with the building blocks for protein as well as with a variety of unsaturated fatty acids and minerals.

■ While you are still in bed, eat some figs or prunes that you have let soak overnight; also, drink the water in which they soaked.

■ You have to count on gaining a couple of pounds (a kilogram) during the recovery days. This amount corresponds roughly to the weight of a full stomach.

The Day Immediately Following the Fast

■ Upon awakening: Figs or prunes soaked in water overnight

■ Breakfast: Two cups of herbal tea or weak black tea

■ During the morning: An apple with the peel and seeds

■ Noon: Potato soup with herbs (see the recipe below)

■ During the afternoon: An apple, herbal tea

■ In the evening: 1¾ oz. (50 g) quark or yogurt with a teaspoon each of linseeds and sandwort juice (sweetened with honey), a slice of melba toast, and herbal tea (for example, balsamic mint or valerian)

Recipe for Potato Soup (One Serving)

Ingredients: A small potato, carrot, leek stalk, celery bulb, parsley stems, half a quart (liter) water, ½ teaspoon oatmeal, some ground nutmeg and marjoram, 1 teaspoon of granulated vegetable broth, and freshly chopped parsley

Preparation: Peel the potatoes, wash the vegetables, and dice. Bring the water to a boil. Place the potatoes

Linseed stimulates the digestive system. In addition, it supplies the entire body with important nutrients.

Tip
After having broken the full fast, you can follow F. X. Mayr's milk-bread fast for two days in order to stimulate the chewing reflex, the saliva, and the stomach secretions. After that, continue with the food recommended for the recovery days.

Grocery List for the Recovery Days

What You May Already Have at Home

Herbal teas, black tea, honey, jelly, onions, sandwort juice (sweetened with honey), linseed, oatmeal, vegetable broth (granulated), seasonings, and lemons

What You May Need to Buy

Melba toast, linseed bread (from a health food store), butter, buttermilk, low-fat quark, low-fat cheese, yogurt, various fruit (including apples, figs, and prunes), nuts, vegetables (including salad ingredients, carrots, fresh herbs, potatoes, leek, celery, and parsley), an egg, and lean ham

---

and the vegetables in the water, and simmer for 20 minutes. Take the soup from the stove, and purée or mash the potatoes and the vegetables with a fork. Add the nutmeg, the marjoram, the oatmeal, and the granulated vegetable broth, as well as some hot water if necessary. Top off with fresh parsley before serving.

Important
Give as much attention now to eating as you just gave to fasting.

The First Recovery Day

■ Upon awakening: Figs or prunes soaked in water overnight

■ Breakfast: Bircher muesli (with apples and nuts, see the recipe on page 69)

■ During the morning: An apple

■ Noon: Salad or a fruit-and-vegetable plate, with potatoes or potato soup (see the soup recipe on page 89)

■ During the afternoon: A slice of melba toast with honey and a cup of herbal tea

■ In the evening: The same as for the afternoon

The Second Recovery Day

■ Upon awakening: A few soaked figs or prunes
■ Breakfast: Bircher muesli, a slice of linseed bread, a piece of melba toast, a small glass of buttermilk, and black tea
■ Noon: Tossed salad, carrots, organic rice, and quark
■ During the afternoon: Buttered melba toast and herbal tea
■ In the evening: A plate of salad, a slice of linseed bread and a piece of melba toast (lightly buttered), low-fat cheese, and herbal tea
■ Throughout the day: Three apples and 12 nuts (such as hazelnuts, walnuts, and cashews)

The Third Recovery Day

■ Upon awakening: A few soaked figs or prunes
■ Breakfast: A slice of linseed bread and a piece of melba toast (buttered and with some jam or honey), perhaps a slice of lean ham, a small glass of buttermilk, and black tea
■ Noon: A plate of fruit and vegetables, a fried egg, and a glass of buttermilk
■ Afternoon: Buttered melba toast with honey and a cup of herbal tea
■ In the evening: A piece of fresh fruit, lightly buttered linseed bread, quark, and herbal tea
■ Throughout the day: Three apples and 12 nuts (such as hazelnuts, walnuts, and cashews)
■ After the last recovery day, you can return to a full nutritional diet.

Eating right—that is, eating moderately—is sometimes more difficult than not eating at all. However, every fast is a chance for a fresh start and an opportunity to break with unhealthy eating practices.

Tip
As you eat your meals, repeat the following three phrases: "I am full" . . . "I've had enough" . . . "I can't eat anymore." The suggestive powers of these phrases will make you feel like eating less.

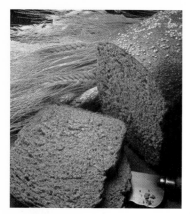

Multigrain products should be a regular part of your diet.

A fast marks a considerable break in one's eating habits. Try not to fall back into the old patterns afterward. Instead, try to adjust yourself, step by step, to new rules for eating. You will soon see what a benefit this has on your health.

The Post-fast Period

Establishing New Eating and Nutritional Habits

Fasting is actually easy. You have probably found this out during the 10-day program. Fasting is certainly easier than eating right and maintaining a healthy diet, especially when you consider all of the tempting foods there are. But you will likely discover that, the more you fast, the more the rules of healthy nutrition will become an inner necessity for you.

So, what is a healthy diet? Opinions vary widely. Take, for instance, the opposing views of vegetarians and meat lovers. There are, however, a few rules that apply to everybody.

Shopping Tips

■ Buy simple, natural, low-fat products. Go out of your way to find fresh fruit and vegetables and meats from organic farms. There, they don't use pesticides on their crops and they care for their animals under proper conditions.

■ You can find good multigrain breads without preservatives at health food stores.

■ Buy fruit and vegetables according to the season from regional farms. Don't buy products that have had to travel from countries far away.

Proper Preparation

■ Don't overcook, because a lot of valuable nutrients are lost during cooking.

■ Use sea salt or full salt with iodine. These salts contain vital trace elements, and they are considerably less detrimental than typical table salt.

■ Use as little salt as possible. Season instead with fresh or dried herbs (such as dill, basil, thyme, oregano, rosemary, and marjoram).

Drinks

■ It's important to drink a lot all the time—not just while you are fasting. Have 2 to 3 quarts, or liters, a day (mineral water, diluted sugar-free fruit juices, and herbal teas).

■ Instead of snacking between meals, try the low-calorie drinks.

■ Coca-Cola and lemonade as well as fruit juices sweetened with sugar should be struck from your list, because they contain too many calories.

■ You should also avoid alcohol, black tea, and coffee.

Meals

■ Eat as healthily as possible.

■ Avoid artificially treated foods, such as sugar and bleached flour, as well as canned, processed, and overcooked foods.

■ Begin each meal with something fresh as an appetizer, such as fruit, salad, or raw vegetables.

You will discover that a proper, nutritional diet reduces the desire for sweets as well as for caffeine and alcohol.

Tip
Organic pasta and brown rice are especially good for our health.

Important
Even fruit yogurt often contains a large amount of sugar. Be sure to read the label.

■ The basis of good nutrition is organic food, especially fruit, vegetables, multigrain products, potatoes, and legumes, as well as milk and milk products.

■ Begin the day with Bircher muesli (see the recipe on page 69) or a whole-grain cereal.

■ Eat meat, sausage, eggs, and fish in moderation.

■ Avoid all pork, and plan one protein-free day a week to keep the body's acid levels normal.

■ Use as little animal fat as possible when cooking; this includes cream, lard, butter, and sour cream. Instead, use a cold-pressed vegetable oil with plenty of unsaturated fatty acids (for example, thistle, soy, olive, or sunflower oil).

■ Avoid sweets that are made with a lot of sugar (cake, candy, cookies, and chocolate). Sweeten instead with honey or a sugar replacement.

Eating Right

■ Eat slowly, and chew thoroughly.

■ Think about what you are eating, without becoming distracted by the television or conversation.

■ Don't eat in a bad mood.

■ Don't overeat. Stop when you begin to feel sated, and leave the rest on your plate.

■ Try not to have dinner any later than 6 P.M. if possible. Keep this adage in mind: "A king in the morning, a pauper in the evening."

■ Turn each meal into a festive event.

■ Plan a letdown day from time to time.

About This Book

About the Authors

Margot Hellmiss is a journalist specializing in the areas of natural healing methods, alternative therapies, and nutrition.

Dr. Norbert Kriegisch is a doctor of natural medicine. He places a great deal of value on a holistic approach to human beings and their health.

A Note to the Reader

This book has been carefully researched and edited. However, its contents are not guaranteed. Neither the authors nor the publisher can be held responsible for possible injury or damage arising from the practical guidelines herein.

Photo Credits

Alfred Pasieka, Hilden: 23; Archive Gerstenberg, Wietze: 11; IFA, Munich 1, 87 (AGE), 20 (Forster), 37 (N.N.), 40 (Tschanz), 47 (E.Pott), 48 (Digu), 50 (Lescourret); Image Bank, Munich: 5 (David de Lossy), 19 (Joseph van Os), 59 (Kaz Mori), 67 (Walter Bibikow), 76 (Francisco Ontanon), 83 (Dann Coffey), 92 (Michael Skott); Tony Stone, Munich: U1 (cover) (Peter Correz); Transglobe, Hamburg: 14 (N.N.), 6 (Jo Clasen)

Index